Finding Your Way Back to YOU

A self-help guide for women who want to regain their Mojo and realise their dreams!

by Lynne Saint

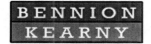

Published by Bennion Kearny Limited
6 Victory House, 64 Trafalgar Road
Birmingham, B13 8BU

www.BennionKearny.com

Cover image: ©Vaclav Volrab

For Jack

About Lynne Saint

Lynne Saint is a professional life coach, author, trainer, hypnotherapist and NLP Master Practitioner. She runs her coaching practice - The Change Coach UK - in Watford, UK.

Lynne is a winner of a National Training Award for her own inspirational self-development, and continues to develop and support others to change their ways of thinking and behaviour - to be the best that they can be.

www.the-change-coach.co.uk

Table of Contents

Introduction

Do you feel that you have been side-tracked from the real **YOU** either by your career, taking time to bring up a family, or being in a relationship? Are you tired of putting others first and always accepting second best? Or do you feel that you have reached a stage in your life where you have become 'stuck', or are at a crossroads, and need some direction.

This book is a practical guide for women of all ages and walks of life, to provide you with the focus, motivation, and new skills and techniques to get you what you really want. It is a resource that you can dip into for reference or strength when you have become the person that you really aspire to be.

It introduces you to new skills that, at first, may seem a bit strange or unfamiliar, but you have already taken the first step to learning new things about yourself - so just go with the flow and enjoy the experience. Each chapter has a similar structure and includes techniques and exercises that will help you to relax and

Introduction

become really focused and motivated on what you want to achieve.

Once you have achieved what you set out to do, this book will be full of your own notes, pictures, reflections and anything else you want to put in it – it's your own personal resource bank and toolkit. You may wish to keep your thoughts and reflections throughout your journey to yourself, and to keep this book in a private place, if that works for you. This is your personal journey to the YOU that you want to be - your own treasure box that will become really special to you as you make progress towards your life goals.

Your journey will not always be an easy ride and I will challenge you to step outside your comfort zone along the way. This represents a serious investment in your time and energy and I will encourage you to reflect regularly and to learn from what challenges you. But don't worry - we will also have a lot of fun and 'a-hah' moments along the way on your journey towards self-discovery!

All of the techniques detailed in this book are free to download from my website, so that you can practice and keep them as your own resource bank whenever you need them. I will never be far away to support you.

Once you start to make progress in changing your behaviour and developing your self-confidence, you may find that some individuals around you will try to railroad you from your path, for a variety of reasons. You might come across 'moodhoovers' or 'energy vampires' who either dismiss or make fun of what you are doing. Steer clear of them and mix with people who encourage, energise and support you, and who will celebrate your successes with you as you make progress towards your new reality.

Alternatively, as you make progress, you may want to share your vision and goals with your partner, friends or family. The choice is yours – remember this is *your* future, so go with your intuition and do what feels right and best for you as you progress and become more confident and self-assured.

Finally, remember that I will be your coach and your biggest supporter and will work with you and guide you to the **YOU** that you really aspire to be. So wherever you are at in your life right now, let's begin the journey!

Lynne

www.the-change-coach.co.uk

Introduction

Throughout this book are various self-reflection boxes and tables to fill in. However, this book is only in A5 size, and space can be a little tight at times. If you are reading an electronic version of the book, filling in the boxes is even more challenging!

Therefore, please feel free to download the accompanying workbook to *Finding Your Way Back to You*.

It contains all the relevant boxes and tables to be filled in. It's nice and big (A4 size) and will make life easier for you.

You can download the PDF file from the Publisher's website:

www.BennionKearny.com/workbook

1

Getting Motivated
Towards YOU

In this chapter we will begin the first steps of your journey towards finding your way back to YOU, by getting all of the energy and motivation you will need to see you through to reaching what you really want. Plus being able to access that energy and motivation, whenever you need it.

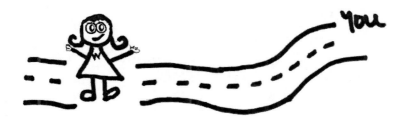

During your journey to YOU, you will learn new ways of managing your behaviour and discover how you can make significant changes to your life. You aren't going to change your unique personality, and neither should you want to, but the new skills that you will learn in this chapter and subsequent chapters will give you the awareness to manage your traits to become your best and most successful self.

Your commitment to yourself

Throughout your journey to the YOU that you really can be, I will be your coach and by working through this workbook will provide you with the skills needed to fulfil your true potential so you can begin to live your ideal life. The vital difference to achieving your full potential is total commitment from you to yourself, and to your goals. This will make all the difference to your success.

So, it's important as you begin your journey, that you understand what this commitment is about, that you truly believe in your own potential and are really willing and motivated to seek a new and fulfilling future for yourself.

Your commitment is made up of the following four elements:

1. Self-belief
2. Motivation
3. Self-discipline
4. Willingness to challenge yourself

Let's look at these four aspects in more detail.

Self-Belief

This is the extent to which you believe - deep inside - that you are worthy and deserve the good things that you will bring to your life. Without self-belief you will sabotage and resist these great things. Your self-belief may just be a small flicker at the moment, but the important thing is that you are willing, with my help, to feel that you are worthy enough to turn the gas up and increase it into a strong flame!

Motivation

This is the most important element of all. Are you sick and frustrated of the direction that your life was going before now? Have you had enough of the insecurities, of feeling second best and overlooked? Have you lost your way? If this describes you and you have had enough of this, and are willing to invest in yourself and do something big about it, then your motivation will be high. Only you know what drives and motivates you personally, so start noticing when you have felt really motivated to do something in the past, and we will work with these positive triggers in future exercises.

Self-Discipline

This is a vital quality to achieving your success, because when the going gets tough 'the tough get going' – and there will be occasions along the way when you will need to give yourself some tough self-talk to get yourself back on track. It will be your self-discipline that keeps you propelled towards your future. It's easy to be energised and enthusiastic when things are going well, but change always brings a certain amount of discomfort and unfamiliarity. There will be days when you don't feel like trying, or when you have a setback; it's these times when you will have to draw on your reserves of courage and determination, so be prepared!

Chapter 1

Willingness to challenge yourself

This is about being willing to challenge yourself and *everything* you know and accept as the status quo in your life. This includes things that you have believed about yourself, and of the world, since childhood. Challenging yourself is necessary to create new ways of thinking and being, and to allow the vast range of new possibilities into your life. If you just stick with what you already know and accept (the familiar) then you will not be open to accept anything new. You will just end up staying where you are – and that's not what you have come this far for, is it?

You will need to suspend your disbelief and *really* believe that the things you want are possible. This will require you to be the best that you can possibly be, and to take responsibility for creating the life that you want. You must want to put the work and effort in, and be prepared to take risks along the way.

So, let's start by looking at your current attitude.

Your attitude – positive or negative?

It's all too easy to blame others for your lot, but until *you* decide to take responsibility for your own situation, then you don't have the power to change it.

If you don't take control or responsibility for your life then someone else will, and sometimes it's just easier for us to allow others to take that control or responsibility, for whatever reason. Unfortunately, this can become the norm in life. We just go with the flow, and agree with the ideas or whims of others, and end up being pretty frustrated or angry with ourselves for not speaking up or making a stand until it's too late.

You might want to ask yourself 'why have I not taken control or responsibility for my life and who I am, before now?' You might already have the answer, and it may be the reason you have started your journey here. Whatever the reason, the past is the past, and you can't change it, but you can change the future and during your journey you will learn new ways of thinking, and techniques which will make you want to change and challenge your behaviour towards an exciting and vibrant future.

Now, we all know people who always seem to be upbeat and in a good mood, no matter what happens to them, or whatever time of the month it is. People whose 'glass is half full'. Are you one of those 'glass half full' people, or do you tend to be of the 'glass half empty' crowd? Do you see the negative in most things, before you consider the positive side, if at all?

Which one are you? The way that you react to situations may be affected by something known as cause and effect.

Are you at currently at cause or effect?

How do you live your life now? At cause, or at effect? It's important to be aware of this distinction. It is rare for any person to *always* live her life at cause; far too many of us live a large portion of our lives at effect - responding to the actions, desires, needs or emotional states of others around us.

Being at cause means that you are in control and have choices in creating what you want in life - you take responsibility for what you have achieved or will achieve. You see the world as a place of opportunity and you move towards achieving what you want. If things are not unfolding as you would like, you take action and explore other possibilities. Above all, you know you have choice in what you do and how you react to people and events. Does this sound like the YOU that you really want to be?

If you are at effect you may blame others or circumstances for your bad moods or for what you have not achieved in general. You may feel powerless or depend on others in order to feel good about yourself or about life. "If only my partner / boss /

Chapter 1

colleagues / parents / children understood me, and helped me achieve my dreams. If only they did what I wanted or what is best for me, then life would be great". Sound familiar?

If you wait around and hope for things to be different, or for others to provide for you, then you are at effect or a victim of circumstance. And really, how much fun is that? How much fun do you think it is for others to be around you? Believing that someone else is responsible, or making them responsible for your happiness (because that's easier for you), for your different moods is very limiting. It gives this person some mystical power over you, which can cause you a great deal of anguish, stress and unhappiness.

Being at cause means you have choices in your life - you can choose what is best for you, while ensuring the choice is ecological for those around you. That is, you consider the consequences of *your* actions on others, but do not take responsibility for *their* emotional well-being. 'Believing' you are responsible for the emotional well-being of someone else can place a heavy burden on you (and can cause a great deal of stress as well).

Those who live their lives at effect often see themselves, or live their lives, as victims with no choices whatsoever. The irony is that they *do* have choice and they have chosen not to choose. Allowing others to control or heavily influence their lives. They have chosen to be responsive to whatever is given to them.

So, if you are currently more at effect, let's get you motivated to be at *cause,* and start making those important changes towards YOU. We'll start by providing you with the mental resources you need to be able to explore positive ways to achieve your goals.

Adopt a Positive Attitude

Whatever personality type you are at the moment, I want you to adopt a positive attitude starting from today. Let's begin by getting an idea of how motivated you are to make those changes towards a positive and exciting future!

How motivated am I?

Ask yourself – on a scale of 1 to 10, with one as the lowest score, how motivated you are today - to finding the YOU that you really want to be.

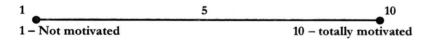

1	5	10
1 – Not motivated		10 – totally motivated

Whatever your score, we want it to be at the higher end of the scale and I'll encourage you to keep measuring it along your journey. Don't worry if it's pretty low or middling at the moment, as we are going to practice some techniques to get you motivated towards YOU. Techniques to use whenever you need a boost!

This exercise uses a technique developed by the Neuro-Linguistic Programming (NLP) pioneers, Richard Bandler and John Grinder, which will help you to reprogram the way you think.

The mind is very sensitive, and as you feel more confident running through this, and future exercises and scenarios in your imagination, you will feel more and more confident in everyday life.

Chapter 1

This is the first of your daily mind workouts, so let's try it. Read it through a few times in advance, so that you know what to do. It might seem a bit strange at first but stick with it. It works! You can use it any time you need to be more motivated and energised.

Daily Workout

The Ring of Motivation and Energy

1. Relax, close your eyes if you need to, and imagine a Ring of Power in front of you on the floor as a circle about 2 feet in diameter. The edges can be any colour you like.

2. Now remember a time when you were totally motivated. Imagine it as a big, bright, focused picture. Remember that feeling, and when you are totally motivated, then step **into** the ring.

3. As soon as the feeling begins to subside, then step **out** of the ring.

4. Now remember a time when you when you felt totally powerful. Imagine it as a big, bright, focused picture. Remember that feeling, and when you are totally powerful then step **into** the ring.

5. As soon as the feeling begins to subside, then step **out** of the ring.

6. Now remember a time when you really felt that you could have whatever you wanted, a time when you could have it all. Imagine it as a big, bright, focused picture. Remember that feeling, and when you could really have it all then step **into** the ring.

7. As soon as the feeling begins to subside, step **out** of the ring.

8. And now remember a time when you really felt really energetic, when you had tons of energy. Imagine it as a big, bright, focused picture. Remember that feeling, and when you could really have it all then step **into** the ring.

9. As soon as the feeling begins to subside, step **out** of the ring.

10. Imagine, taking the Ring of Power from the floor and squeezing it smaller. Until it's small enough to fit on your finger and slip it on.

Whenever you feel you need more energy or you are lacking in motivation, simply concentrate for a few moments, put on your ring, and access your inner motivation and energy stores.

Repeat this simple exercise at least once a day, or listen to the weblink at *www.the-change-coach.co.uk* every day for a week and you will allow yourself to move further towards the YOU that you want to be.

Now, that you have completed the exercise, on a scale of 1 to 10, how motivated are you to find the YOU that you want to be? If you are not a lot higher on the scale than before, keep practicing and you will get more motivated and energised the more you do it.

Daily Visualisation

This technique is all about starting to create a picture or a movie of what your future will look like. I will help you to clarify your direction and goals in future chapters as you progress. So for this exercise, just go with your imagination!

Repeat this simple exercise at least once a day, or (as above) listen to the weblink at *www.the-change-coach.co.uk* every day for a week, and you will allow yourself to move further towards the YOU that you want to be.

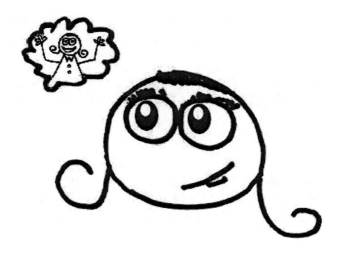

Dreaming yourself to the future YOU

1. Take a few moments to relax; close your eyes and breathe deeply.

2. Continue to breathe in through your nose to a count of seven, and breathe out to a count of eleven, pushing all of the air out of your lungs as you breathe out. (If you can't manage seven/eleven, breathe to as many counts as is comfortable, but ensure you breathe out more than you breathe in).

3. Now, when you breathe in - imagine the air is a beautiful, vibrant colour, and then imagine the same colour much, much more faded as you breathe out. You have breathed in all of the wonderful, life energising air and absorbed all of its goodness and breathed out what's left.

4. As your muscles relax, it becomes easier and easier to unleash your imagination.

5. Now, imagine another you standing in front of you, having achieved your goal or goals.

6. Take a moment to feel totally elated with the YOU that you set out to be.
    Look at the way she stands, shoulders back with real, tangible confidence. Notice the way she smiles, beams even, how she walks, how she talks. Look at her hairstyle, the stylish clothes that suit her, just right. Notice how she speaks to others, how she handles problems and how she simply goes for it!

7. Now, step into your confident self.
    See through her eyes, hear through her ears, and feel how it feels *sooo* good to live life as YOU.

8. Take a minute to daydream about how your life will be different as you live more and more as YOU.

Now, write down in the following box - or in your downloaded workbook - what you 'imagined' as the future YOU, or draw a picture or paste pictures in from a magazine – what do you look like, feel like, where are you, who are you with?

Chapter 1

What do you look like, feel like, where are you, who are you with?

The Future Me

If it makes it more real for you, consider creating a poster sized collage of all of the parts that will make YOU. These can be words and cuttings from magazines that represent your future for you. Whichever way you choose (you are already controlling your choices to YOU!), make them big, bold and colourful, and put them somewhere you will see them regularly. Really go for it!

You have now started to form a real picture of what the real YOU looks, sounds, and feels like when you have achieved everything you set out to do on your journey, and you are totally motivated to achieve that. To maintain your positive attitude, you will need to practice your new ways of thinking and the above techniques every day. They will force you into a much richer, positive state of mind and new ways of thinking

It's important that you revisit your picture, either on the page above, or by having it prominently displayed somewhere where you will see it regularly. Replay the short 'YOU' movie that you imagined in this chapter, regularly. Find ways that keep you motivated towards what makes it real for you, so revisit your thoughts, your drawing, or your picture every day. Remember keep it real and regular!

If you always do what you have always done, you will always get the same result, so do it differently.

Me Time

You may wish to allocate a time and a space each day to just be by yourself… to think back on the day and at what you have achieved.

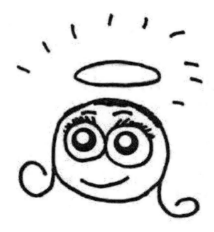

Our whole dynamic system is one of highs and lows, activity and recovery. Taking time out to look after ourselves makes us better able to function effectively. A ten minute pause allows us to reduce stress hormones and lets our bodies and minds return to equilibrium. You might want to play some relaxing music, light scented candles, or just enjoy the silence.

In the time it takes for you to have some 'Me' time, you are able to get back to YOU, and become ready for the next challenge of the day.

Feeling guilty about investing in yourself? In starting your journey or taking time out for 'Me' time? Do you describe yourself as selfless in your everyday life? Remember that you are not a martyr and you are truly worth the investment in yourself!

If putting yourself first is a significant change for you, this may help. Think of the safety advice on an airplane – the emergency procedure instructs you to place a mask over your own face before trying to help another person. This should be a metaphor for your own life. If you look after yourself, you will be better able to attend to the needs of others. So, never feel guilty, take regular time out to enjoy the moment. Those little things that delight and make you feel good about yourself can be healing and uplifting when you systematically include them in your daily routine.

'Me' time will help you to recharge your batteries, give you time to reflect and think things through and to plan ahead. Mostly it will allow you to relax and clear your thoughts.

Time to look back... but only for a while!

You can lift your spirits by writing down your positive thoughts and opening your mind to exciting possibilities. You'll feel instantly energised by the first steps to self-discovery you have started to make, and the prospect of great things coming your way.

Write down any changes in your behaviour, feelings or ways of thinking since you have started your journey – nothing is too small or insignificant. Small steps are just fine and they might not be many, but keep adding to the list as they occur to you.

Chapter 1

Remember, this is all about reflecting and learning from events and experiences. It's not about dwelling on the past; it's about looking back, learning from it and moving forward with new knowledge that you can use it to your advantage in the future.

Reflections / Changes I have noticed already

Give yourself a pat on the back for what you have achieved so far. Give thanks and gratitude for all of the skills, inner resources and the people in your life, and all of the good things that you already have that make you happy. Look out to the future with a positive attitude, to what you will continue to achieve as a confident, happy and fulfilled woman. See what she sees, hear how she speaks, feel what she feels... and smile!

Daily Checklist towards YOU

Tick these off as you achieve and practice them:

Done Daily Workout and tried on the Ring of Motivation & Energy	
Practised being motivated and energised	
Done Daily Visualisation	
Revisited my 'YOU' movie and completed my picture of the future me	
Had 'Me' time	
Written down changes I've already noticed about myself	
Given thanks and gratitude for what I already have	

Summary

Well done! You have already taken the brave and courageous first steps on your personal path. You now have some new skills in your personal resource bank that you can practice in order to motivate and energise yourself to achieve so much more.

Chapter 1

You've already started to develop a picture, both in your mind and in this book (or even on your wall) of your future, and you've begun to take valuable 'Me' time to reinforce this image. You are investing time in yourself, without feeling guilty about it and you have started to notice the changes in yourself and ways of thinking that will steadily increase as your journey continues.

Remember, if you think differently, you will feel differently - and what you can achieve is limitless. So, now that you have caught your breath, let's move on!

It's never too late to be what you might have been

George Elliott, Author

2

Getting Rid of the Old Stuff

In this chapter we will work together to help you to identify any self-made barriers or obstacles that may be preventing you from moving forward from the past. I will challenge you to take a close look at your existing behaviours, and limiting beliefs, and decisions.

We will explore and tackle why you think about your limiting beliefs, why you are still holding on to them, and identify which ones are holding you back from achieving what you have set out to do. We will then work on ways to change your old ways of thinking, towards your new, more compelling future.

Chapter 2

Limiting Beliefs

Limiting beliefs can be described as negative beliefs that we hold about ourselves and other people. Our limiting beliefs create internal mental chatter which is self-deprecating and imposes limitations on what we allow ourselves to do. In other words, they hold us back and restrict our lives.

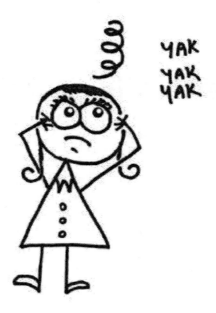

Stress, anxiety, a lack of confidence and even depression can evolve from these limiting belief 'mind tapes' that play over and over in our heads, and form a habitual way of negative thinking.

Any time that you have adopted or accepted a limiting belief such as 'I'm not good enough' or 'I'm too fat', you made a limiting decision *before* that belief became real for you. In other words, *you chose* to believe something was true. This will continue to remain a reality for you until you challenge this way of thinking.

In the table below - or in your workbook - I want you to list your own limiting beliefs that could potentially be holding you back from trying new ways of being. These are thoughts that are usually preceded with:

- "I could never…"
- "I don't have time to…"
- "I wouldn't…"

In the left hand column, write down all of your limiting beliefs that come to mind. Keep coming back and adding to this list as you think of them.

In the middle column, write down when you decided each limiting belief to be true of you.

Then, in the right hand column, write down a comment that was made by another person, or the event or situation that contributed to you choosing to make this limiting decision into a belief.

Chapter 2

Limiting Belief (what you believe you can't do)	When did you decide this?	Event or Comment
e.g. 'I'm not clever'	e.g. 'When I was 11 years old'	e.g. 'I failed my 11 plus exam and my dad said I was stupid'

Why should I change my self-limiting beliefs?

By changing your self-limiting beliefs and becoming more aware of your behaviour and how you project yourself to others, you will be removing one of the major obstacles in your way to transforming yourself into the person that you aspire and want to be. Self-confidence can be built by simply changing your beliefs about your abilities, skills, and full potential.

You have already taken the first steps to changing your old ways of behaviour, as you have consciously admitted that you have limiting beliefs in the exercise above.

The hardest and most important step in changing your beliefs, and your behaviour as a result, involves proving exactly the opposite of the belief by going against it. It's not as easy as it sounds and the changes won't happen overnight, as it has taken many years to establish the old way of thinking into a self-fulfilling habit.

The Power of having a Positive Outlook

Remember, you are starting to break a long established habit of negative and limiting beliefs here, so you will need to recognise the effects that they have on you, and keep correcting yourself every time a self-limiting belief pops into your mind.

Every time a self-limiting belief enters your thoughts, I want you to ask yourself the following questions:

1. 'Is it true?'

2. 'How do I usually react when my mind thinks a self-limiting belief?'

Chapter 2

Notice your change in mood, in confidence? Does your facial expression change? Does your voice sound different when you respond to a question with 'I can't...'? How do you feel inside?

The more you become conscious of the effect that self-limiting beliefs have on you, the more you can begin to start challenging your old ways of thinking.

So, how do you change your self-limiting beliefs, and your negative 'mind tapes', and the effect they have on you and your life right now?

You may have heard of the phrase: 'there is no failure, only feedback'. Many successful people experience lots of failures before they eventually became a success. The difference in them, compared to those who don't succeed, is that every time something didn't work out as planned, they learned from the experience, made some adjustments and tried again, until they did achieve what they wanted.

You may want to revisit some memories which you previously thought were failures with your new positive perspective, and note the learning or lessons that you can now take with you, into the future, which you may have not previously noticed.
It may be that you didn't get into a particular school as a child and have viewed this as a failure ever since. Go back and reframe the experience: consider the friends that you made, or the teachers that made a difference, that you would never have met, if you had succeeded in your original plan.

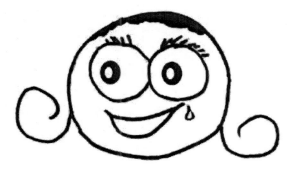

I'm sure you can think of many experiences when if you hadn't done X then you would never have done Y! Don't forget to focus on the positives and not on your old ways of thinking.

Write them down here and keep adding to them as your positive outlook gets stronger with practice!

Event or Experience	Positive things that I learned from it

You will need to constantly challenge your negative thoughts every time you hear one in your head, until your unconscious mind gets the message that you can do whatever you thought you couldn't do previously.

You will need to be aware that you may start off with thoughts similar to 'I can't...' so just rephrase your internal dialogue to 'I used to think that... but now I can...' and keep behaving as if you have followed this behaviour forever – *Act the part!* Act as if you have always been a positive, confident person.

With practice the new, positive behaviour that follows these positive thoughts will come naturally, and those old negative habits will be replaced by new, positive ones. Notice the great feelings of achievement!

Turning Down the Volume of Your Inner Critic or Wimp!

We all have an inner critic, or inner wimp, that is our own worst enemy, and which constantly restricts our behaviours. We weren't born with these behaviours - we have learned them over many years, from our parents, family, friends and other influential people in our lives. This internal dialogue is not easy to turn down and it does take practice as you've already realised.

However, no matter how much you have struggled in the past, we are now concentrating on creating your ideal future, so stay with it. You already have the resources you need to succeed; you just need to recognise them, polish them up, and channel them to achieve what you really want. Every moment of every day provides you with opportunities to make new choices and to practice being the YOU that you know you can be.

So if you were tuned into your old dull, negative internal radio station, now is the time to retune your mind radio onto a more upbeat, positive station. *Turn up the volume!*

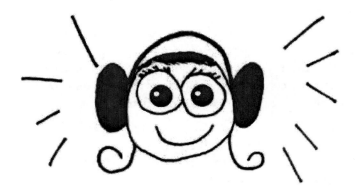

Daily Workout

The next exercise is a great tool to practice when you are lacking in willpower, or when your inner critic or wimp is getting the better of you. We have already seen that the more we repeat a pattern of behaviour, the stronger that pattern of behaviour becomes.

You are now going to practice interrupting that learned pattern of negative behaviour. So, for the next few weeks, whenever you feel negative about anything, or you feel your willpower to succeed is waning, I want you to stop what you are doing and follow the following five steps:

1. Ask yourself *what* you are feeling negative about and notice the picture, or sounds or the feelings that come to mind.
    As you see the picture in your mind, notice:
    - Is it in colour or black and white?

- Where is it located? Is it in front of you? Is it to the left or right?
- Is it big or small?
- Is it a movie, or is it still?
- Is it focussed or fuzzy?
- Is there any sound?

2. Your emotions are like signals or warnings to alert you to possible outcomes. For example, you might feel anxious about a particular situation. Your mind is alerting you to the possibilities of what might go wrong so that you can prepare yourself in advance. Ask yourself now that you are aware, *what* is the message the emotion you are experiencing wants to give you?

3. Act on the message your mind is giving you and make a mental list of every possible scenario; you will be prepared to take action on at least one, if not more of them.
Take a few moments to think of some ways that you can *solve* these problems.

4. Turn off the inner critic or wimp, just like you would press the delete button on your computer. Drain all colour out of your mental picture, shrink it and ping it off into the distance, as if it's attached to an elastic band. If it reappears, ask yourself if there was anything you missed, then just drain the colour out again, shrink it down and ping it away again.

5. Finally, take a few moments to imagine your life as you ideally want it to be. What would you really like to do? With whom, and where? What would you most like to have?

Chapter 2

Next up is another technique to practice every time a negative thought pops into your head. You will reap the benefits through sheer repetition and by challenging your way of thinking until you recondition your mind. You will continue to be positive, energised, and start getting a real zest for life and for what's ahead of you.

Daily Visualisation

Read through the exercise a couple of times so that you are comfortable with it, and take a few moments to relax and breathe deeply. Let your muscles relax and it will be easier to go with the flow of your imagination.

New Belief Generator

1. Choose a belief that you want to have. Now imagine, standing in front of you, 'another you'. A *you* that already has the *belief* that you want to make your own.

2. Now, imagine what it feels like having that belief, which enables 'that other you' to be whatever you want to be. As an example here, let's choose 'I am extremely confident'. Is that other you already extremely confident?

3. Imagine that other you demonstrating this belief. How does the other you behave? How would it feel to have this belief? How does she feel? What does the other you say? What does her voice sound like? How does she walk? How does she dress?

4. If you are not sure yet, pretend how you think it would be. If it isn't quite how you want it to be, make some adjustments, change what needs to be changed to make you feel better. Allow your imagination to be your guide.

When you are happy with the other you, step into her. See what she sees, hear what she hears, and feel what she feels.

5.   When you are ready to step back into your own self - bring *with you* the good feelings, the things you have learned, the new perspective and the new belief.

6.   Now think of a situation that you would like to view from your new outlook. Think through what it is like to have that new outlook, all of the (in our example) confidence you could ever need. How different are things going to be? How different will you feel?

7.   For the next few weeks, act or pretend that your new belief is true. Even if it feels unfamiliar, it will teach you to live more and more as your true self in any number of situations in the future.

Repeat these simple exercises at least once a day, or listen to the weblinks at *www.the-change-coach.co.uk* every day for a week. As you do, you will allow yourself to move further towards the YOU that you know you can be.

Moodhoovers and Energy Vampires

As touched upon in the Introduction, there will be certain people in your life who constantly drain you of energy, and who put you instantly into a negative mood when in their company. They are usually selfish, self-centred individuals who you listen to out of politeness; their sapping of your time and energy has just become a habit for both of you. But it is a constant cycle that you need to break free of and conserve your energies to move forwards and invest in your progress.

Now is the time to recognise what they give you (or don't) and escape. Don't let them near and avoid their company at all cost! Be brave and interrupt this habitual pattern of behaviour – you may find that as you begin to develop into the more confident positive YOU that you feel that you no longer have so much in common with these individuals.

Don't feel guilty about letting go of the Moodhoovers and Energy Vampires in your life. These may be the very people that have kept you back all this time. The time *before* you began to see the real YOU, and the future that you want for yourself.

If this is how you feel - associate with people that give you a lift and make you feel energised and appreciated.

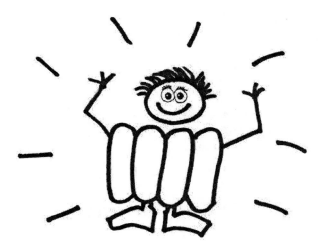

It might help to list your personal 'Energy Radiators' below and make plans to be with them some more. Note also, the Moodhoovers and Energy Vampires that you plan to avoid.

Be aware that you will need to keep practicing your positive outlook and be aware of your own behaviour when in their company - and not become a Moodhoover or Energy Vampire to them!

Remember – *practice makes perfect!*

Your new ways of thinking and behaving will take some practice. After all, you have been practising your old ways of behaviour for years! It's just like when you do a new exercise, your muscles ache until you keep flexing them and they get used to exercise. Exercise becomes easier and enjoyable the more you do it. Simple!

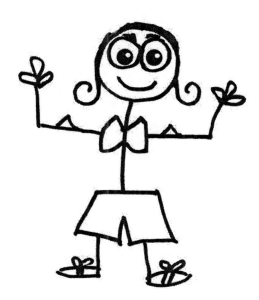

Chapter 2

Energy Radiators versus Moodhoovers and Energy Vampires

Moodhoovers and Energy Vampires in my life	Energy Radiators

Me Time

How's the 'Me' time going? Are you setting aside regular times for yourself to relax and reflect on your achievements? If you are used to putting others first, this may take you some time to get used to, but this is an important aid to your progress.

During 'Me' time, over the next few weeks, I want you to think of all of the things you have meant to do, or experience, where the old you either stopped yourself or you just didn't get around to it. If it helps you to remember, write them down and keep adding to your list as you think of them.

If your previous automatic response to new ideas - "I'm too busy" or "I haven't got the time" – sounds familiar, well, that was the old negative you and now is the time to start practicing your new positive skills. Just like the previous technique, it will be unfamiliar at first, just like when you start exercising certain muscles after a long spell of inertia. The muscles will be aching or even painful at first, but the more you do, the easier the exercise is, and the more toned and strong the muscle becomes. So let's start flexing your muscles of positivity!

As well as practising your exercises on the previous pages, I want you to start trying out new things. It can be anything – small or huge and doesn't have to cost anything except your time.

Stretch your imagination and say to yourself 'why not?!?' should your inner critic or wimp try to resurface for a minute. Try reading a different newspaper for a few days, retune to another radio or TV channel. Go to your local park or museum, check out your local library, or start a short course at your local college. Shop somewhere else, look up friends that you have been meaning to see for ages or have lost touch with. Starting with small, manageable steps will give you the impetus to think bigger. Just go for it and just experience something outside of your comfort zone.

Be your own tourist and take in the world outside your front door. You might not like everything you try, but you will be opening yourself up to lots of new experiences and discoveries, some of which you can grow and take forward with you, into your future.

The important thing is to keep giving it a go. You will never know whether you might enjoy it, you might just surprise yourself! If you don't try, you will never know!

Time to Reflect and celebrate your progress so far

Write down any changes in your behaviour, feelings or ways of thinking since you have started this chapter – don't forget, *nothing is too small or insignificant*. Small steps are just fine and there might not be many, but keep adding to the list as they occur to you, as you continue to recognise your achievements along the way.

Reflections / Changes I have noticed

Daily Checklist towards YOU

Tick these off as you achieve and practice them:

Listed my self-limiting beliefs	
Challenged my limiting beliefs with the two questions	
Completed my list of events or experiences with a positive attitude	
Done my Daily Workout	
Done my Daily Visualisation	
Continued to practice 'Me' time	
Written down changes I've already noticed	
Given thanks and gratitude for the resources and skills that I already have	

Summary

Go Girl! Wow – what changes already!

You will be starting to get used to challenging your old self-limiting beliefs and will have started to recognise the changes in your behaviour as a result of this.

You will have started to step outside of your comfort zone and are beginning to get used to the exercises and techniques that will change the way you think, and ultimately the way in which you behave in the future.

Those around you will also start to notice the changes in you, if they haven't already done so. Your new confidence and positive attitude will have a profound impact on the speed at which you will now start to progress towards the goals that we will work together to set, in the next chapter. You have already laid the first stepping stones to your continued success.

"

Be vigilant, guard your mind against negative thoughts

Buddha

"

3

Reality Check
where are you now?

In this chapter I will introduce you to more tools and techniques which may be new to you. They will help you to reflect and assess all the areas of your life as they are right now. These reflections and assessments will help you judge what areas of your life are taking up most of your time and what areas are being neglected.

You can then decide on your priority areas and the people in them that are most important to you and those that require more attention from you. You can then focus more resources into those areas to move in the right direction, without having your energy sapped in areas that are neither beneficial nor part of your journey towards your exciting future.

Chapter 3

Auditing Your Life

No matter what stage you are in your life right now, it's always a good idea to take a stock check or audit and to appreciate all that you have achieved so far, and all of the skills that you already possess.

It makes sense to evaluate where you currently stand before you take the next step - making your new future a reality. You will then have an idea of how near (or far) you are to achieving it, and this will help you to plan properly and structure your plans into positive, manageable steps.

I want you to imagine your life with you - as you are today - at the centre of it, with your past stretching out behind you, and your future in front of you. Alternatively, imagine your past and future however best works for you. Up, down, sideways - it doesn't matter.

I have included an example of this, below, to help you.

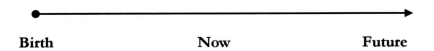

Birth   **Now**   **Future**

Now, on your own time line, I want you to remember back and visualise all of the positive (and only the positive) significant events that have made you the person that you are today.

Close your eyes and take a few deep breaths if it's easier to remember that way. Take your time.

Now, on the table below, list all of the *significant events* where you learned or noticed a particular skill or attribute that you have. It could be a time when you really handled a situation well, or succeeded at something that you had really strived for, maybe an exam or a target that you had set yourself?

List these on the right hand side of the box below, then on the left hand side, list all of the actual *positive* attributes and skills that you have gained from those events, which you can now acknowledge are great skills and take forward with you into the future.

Use more paper if you need to and staple it to this page for future reference, or use the downloadable workbook

This is an opportunity to blow your own trumpet and you may not be used to doing it. So don't dismiss anything, write it down. No one is judging you, so include anything that you feel is worth mentioning – there are no rights or wrongs.

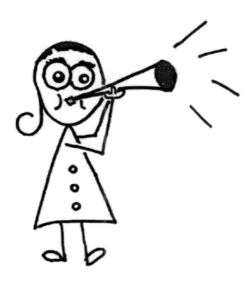

Your personal CV - Now

Significant Event	Skills and Attributes
e.g. started school/college/university, travelled abroad, gained qualifications, met ??, got married, passed driving test, had children, etc	*e.g. I can drive, I have patience, experience in, I am a qualified (name job), I am patient, etc*

Now, take a moment to reflect on all that you have. Give thanks to yourself and all of those significant people in your life that helped you to achieve your skills.

Be grateful for all of those special attributes that make you unique, that you can utilise and take forward with you, whilst you continue to grow towards the woman you want to be.

Now the fun part! You have already acknowledged the skills that you will take with you to your future, now I want you write down the skills and attributes that you would *like to develop* for the future.

It might help to think of people or attributes that you admire or role models and their qualities that you have had in the past or have in your life now.

Your personal CV – Future Skills I want to Develop

Skills I want to Develop	What will this do for me?
e.g. Learn to drive, speaking confidently, learn to swim, patience, etc	*e.g. Make me independent, make me less anxious in company, spend more time with the kids, make me more calm, etc*

You have now identified all of your positive skills and attributes, and the ones that you want to develop, so now can we move on to the areas of your life that we need to work on and start making YOU a reality?

When life is busy, or all of your energy is focused on a special task that needs to be done and it is all absorbing, it's all too easy to find yourself 'off balance' and not paying enough attention to other important areas of your life. You prioritise what needs to be done and become aware of all of the other things that are being neglected or which require your attention – later – when the most immediate tasks are finished.

While you need to have drive and focus - if you're going to get things done, taking this too far can lead to frustration and intense stress and even guilt that you have neglected a certain person or task that has had to take a back seat for a time.

That's when it is time to take a 'helicopter view' of your life, so that you can bring things back into balance, reduce your anxiety and stress, and begin to turn down the volume of your inner critic and regain control.

Chapter 3

The Wheel of Life

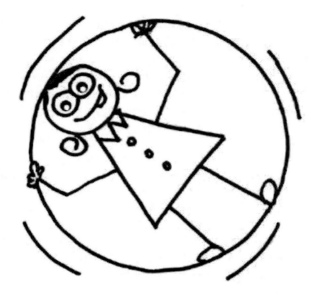

Commonly used by professional life coaches, the Wheel of Life (or Life Wheel) helps you consider each area of your life in turn and assess what's off balance. And so, it helps you to identify areas that need more attention, but feel free to change these headings to suit your own life. Or use the accompanying workbook.

The figure below the following exercise shows a Wheel of Life with example dimensions, or areas of your life, that could be important to you.

1. Start by brainstorming the 6 to 8 areas of your life that are important for you. Different approaches to this are:

- **The roles you play in life,** for example:
  wife/partner, mother/daughter/grandmother,
  manager, colleague, team member, sports
  player, volunteer, or friend.

  or

- **Areas of life that are important to you,**
  for example: career, education, family, friends,
  financial freedom, physical challenge, pleasure,
  artistic expression, positive attitude, or public
  service.

  or

- **Your own combination of these (or
  different) things,** reflecting the things that are
  your most important priorities in life.

2. Write down these areas on the Wheel of Life diagram
    below and cross out and amend them if yours are
    different from the example. Put a different area of
    importance to you in each section of the Life Wheel.

3. This approach assumes that you will be happy and
    fulfilled if you can find the right balance of attention for
    each of these areas. Different areas of your life will need
    different levels of attention, at different times. So the
    next step is to *assess* the amount of attention you're
    currently devoting to each area.

4. Consider each area of your life in turn, and on a scale of
    0 (low) to 10 (high), write down the amount of attention
    you're devoting to that area of your life now. Remember
    to give each section a score between 0-10 and feel free

to add areas if they are not covered below; it's just an example to get you thinking.

5. Does your Life Wheel look and feel balanced? Have you identified areas that you feel *should* be receiving more attention from you and some that are getting *more* attention but shouldn't?

6. Next it's time to consider your ideal level in each area of your life. A balanced life does not mean getting 10 in each life area: some areas need more attention and focus than others at any time. And inevitably you will need to make choices and compromises, as your time and energy are not in unlimited supply!

7. So the question is - what would the ideal level of attention be for you in each life area?

8. Only you can answer this one, but you might like to give each area on the wheel a different score for the level of attention you would like to devote to that area, from now on and in the future. For example, you might like to write this new score in a different colour beside the existing one. So if you have already given the area of 'family/partner' a score of 5, and want to increase it to a score of 8, then write 5/8 and so forth, in each section of your wheel. Your future scores are the areas where you would like to give more attention and these will become the basis of your plan of action.

9. Now you have a visual representation of your current life balance and your ideal life balance. What are the changes in your scores? These are the areas of your life that need attention.

10. And remember that scores can go both ways. There are almost certainly areas that are not getting as much attention as you'd like. However there may also be areas where you're putting in more effort than you'd ideally like to. These areas are sapping energy and enthusiasm

that may be better directed elsewhere. So try to be objective and honest on the areas that are really taking up all of your time and energy.

My Life Wheel

The attention I am currently devoting to each of the important areas of my life:

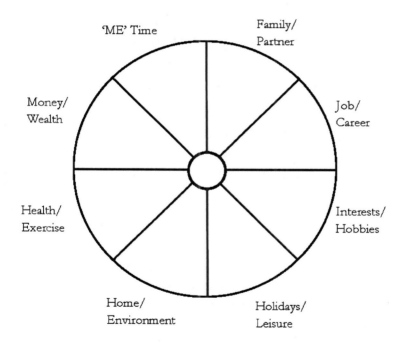

The Wheel of Life is a great tool to help you improve your life balance. It helps you quickly and visually identify the areas in your life to which you want to devote more energy, and helps you to identify and understand where you might want to cut back.

The challenge now is to transform this knowledge and desire for a more balanced life into a positive plan of action that you will need to work on, to regain balance in your life, which we will do more of in the next chapter.

 You have used the Wheel of Life to help identify the areas you want to work on and you can see that it is a great way of visualising your current and your desired life. Once you are working on improving your life balance, it's also a useful tool for monitoring your life balance as it changes over time.

So keep revisiting your completed wheel of life and note down the changes in the scores, and keep a track of the changes as you make progress towards your new, focussed future.

Write down on the table below your current and ideal scores in the areas of your life that are important to you. I've left room at the bottom for you to add more if you need to.

Regaining Balance

	Areas of my Life that are most Important to Me	Current Score	Future Score
1	Family/Partner		
2	Job/Career		
3	Money/Wealth		
4	Health/Exercise		
5	Home/Environment		
6	Holidays/Leisure/Social Life		
7	Interests/Hobbies		
8	ME Time		
9	Other (give name)		
10	Other (give name)		

Let's move on. Starting with the neglected areas, what things do you need to start doing to regain balance in your life?

In the areas that currently sap your energy and time, what can you STOP doing or reprioritise or even delegate to someone else? Make a commitment to these actions by writing them down below in My Life Action Plan.

Note: for the purposes of the book, the columns are pretty narrow, so feel free to copy the plan and make it your own with colours, wider columns and different fonts so that it becomes real and visual for you. Alternatively, use the accompanying workbook which is downloadable at *www.the-change-coach.co.uk* This could be another addition to your wall!

My Life Action Plan

Important Areas of my Life that need my attention:
(Insert from list above starting with the one that's most important and that needs your attention urgently)

What do I need to do?	How will I do it?	Who can help me?	What resources do I need?	When will I achieve it?	How will I know if I have achieved it?

Repeat your Life Action Plan for *each* of the areas that you identified on your Life Wheel, until you have covered them all and have actions to achieve for all of them.

Daily Workout

Have you ever experienced that amazing state of mind when time seems to go into slow motion and you are able to do, or say, just the right thing at the right moment? A situation comes up and you handle it like a dream? You are thinking clearly, you're alert, and you are relaxed and quietly confident?

Some people call this feeling as being in the 'zone', or in the 'now'.

When you are in the zone, you do what you do fantastically well, with a greater sense of control and ease. Some athletes at the top of their sport describe this feeling, but you may have experienced it to a lesser degree doing something you excel at.

If you get into this state when you are focussed on making your plans a reality, you'll not only find that your ideas flow more easily but you will also be able to access your inner resources and use them to your advantage – effortlessly!

Here is a simple exercise that will enable you, with practice, to be able to trigger this state of mind any time you need to.

Creating More Resources for Yourself

Read the exercise all the way through before you begin.

1. Relax and take some deep breaths, and close your eyes if it's easier for you.
    Now, vividly remember a time when you were in the

zone, doing something you love doing. This could be laughing out loud with friends, swimming, dancing, being totally focussed on something – anything, it doesn't matter. Anything you were doing when you felt totally in control with everything going perfectly.

2. Keep going through that memory again and again until you begin to feel that you are in the 'zone' state of mind.

3. When you do, and when you feel the sensation is at its peak, squeeze the thumb and middle finger of your left hand together.

4. Continue to keep reliving this memory in your mind. As you get the zone feeling at its peak continue to squeeze the thumb and middle finger of your left hand together. While you are in the zone, imagine yourself achieving all of the goals that you have set yourself, easily and effortlessly. See yourself handling any obstacles along the way effortlessly and with confidence.

5. Whenever you need to get into the zone state of mind in the future, simply squeeze you thumb and middle finger of our left hand together to access these inner resources.

We practised exercising your new beliefs in the previous chapter, so now that you have been living your new beliefs for a little while and have been recording the changes in this workbook, here is technique to help you to practice the new behaviours that you have started to use, with all of your new knowledge about yourself.

Daily Visualisation

New Behaviour Generator

STEP 1: Select the behaviour worth having.

1. Identify a wanted behaviour: think of the behaviour that you would like to exhibit, or one that you would like to improve upon.
2. Specify context: identify when and where you would like to demonstrate this behaviour.
3. Identify your role model: think of someone you know who behaves in this way. It could be a friend, a fictional person, a film star, or even a member of your own family. It does not matter if you know this person personally, you can pretend. It is only important that you have a good representation of your chosen role model behaving in a way that you would like to behave yourself.
4. Evaluate your Role Model: now run a mental movie of your role model behaving in the way that you would like to in certain situations. Pay attention to their facial expressions, posture, and the words they use, voice, tone, tempo, volume, and pay attention to the response this person gets from people around them.

STEP 2: Replace your Role Model with Yourself and Evaluate

Now I would like you to play that movie again but this time instead of seeing your role model behaving the way that you want to, I want you to see yourself behaving this way, just as your role model did it. As you are doing this make any adjustment you feel you would like to. Take all the time you need.

Do you like the feelings you get from the movie you just watched? Repeat the movie until you get good feelings when running the movie in your mind.

STEP 3: Associate into the New Behaviour

Okay, what I would like you to do now is to run that movie again and as you begin to run it - step inside it and imagine yourself behaving in your chosen manner. See what you would actually be seeing, hear what you would actually be hearing, including the sound of your own voice, and feel what you would actually be feeling. Make sure you really feel your body as you engage in your new behaviour.

Take all the time you need.

Did you enjoy your new behaviour? Is it still something that you would like to be able to do? If yes, go on to the next step. If no, go back to step 2. And repeat until you do.

STEP 4: Future Pace and Test

Now find a situation in the near future when it will be appropriate or desirable to exhibit this behaviour. Run a movie of yourself in that situation using your new behaviour. Step into that movie and directly experience what it would be like to behave that way and in that situation. Make any adjustment that will improve your performance.

As you comfortably continue this process, your unconscious mind is recording your new behaviour in the deepest part of your unconscious mind so that this becomes a permanent part of your unconscious and a permanent part of your everyday life.

That's not because I say so, it's simply because that's just the way it is… isn't it?

Repeat these exercises at least once a day, or listen to the weblink at *www.the-change-coach.co.uk* and you will be pleasantly surprised at how much your life changes from this moment on.

Me Time

Are you still managing to fit your 'Me' time in now that you are so energized and focused on your future?

If this is still something you are struggling with, remember that you don't need permission to take 'Me' time. Don't wait for it, just do it!

The plans you make for yourself are as important as anything that might keep you from them. Keep track. Start to build up to an hour-plus a day. The time can be snatched in ten minute intervals if that fits with your life better.

The important thing is that you do take it, and make time for yourself regularly. Experiment in finding ways to nurture time that can best benefit you. Perhaps during one week, plan two or three hours in one day and skip the next day. See what suits you best.

Chapter 3

Above all else, do not feel guilty! 10% of your time, spent as 'Me time' leaves 90% for others. Be sure to take your full 10% each week!

Women often get caught in the trap of feeling indispensable. We tend to be a bit of a mother hen and want to oversee and do everything. We don't have it all - we do it all. But we have to learn to feel comfortable about occasionally being unavailable to others. It's not healthy to 'be there' all the time - not for a spouse/partner, a child, a friend, a parent or a job. We must concentrate more on being there for ourselves on a regular basis. We can never guarantee to others that we will always be there for them. After all, life throws us numerous surprises, things happen, and our plans do not always work out as we want them to. On the other hand, we can assure our availability to ourselves in most cases. All we can do for others is *try our best*.

We worry about not being perfect. When we can't meet our own unrealistic expectations, we feel discouraged and demoralised. The ideal of perfection can be dangerous to your personal well-being and keeps you from living to the fullest potential. We are all human. Strive, persist, and then relax and live with the knowledge that you have done your best. Expect some problems so that you will not be disappointed when they come. If you lower your expectations, you will be happier in the reality of the moment. If you don't expect to be perfect, you are more likely to experiment, improvise, and take risks. You are more likely to have fun! Once you eliminate the idea of perfection, and retain the idea of being the best that you can be, you will lose your fear of trying new things. And when you lower your expectations, while making sure always to nurture yourself, nothing can hold you back.

Remember that all the time spent looking after yourself will enrich and strengthen your time and your relationships with others. That is the secret to your success and happiness, and now that you have started, you will have set yourself on a path that will lead to your new exciting future and contentment.

Time to Reflect and Celebrate your progress so far

Continue to write down any changes in your behaviour, feelings or ways of thinking since you started this chapter. Note down your energy levels, and the impact that taking 'Me' time is having on yourself and others in your life.

What impact has rebalancing your time and energy had (or started to have) on the important aspects of your life? Has anyone commented on your new behaviour? Was this positive, and if not - what do you think their reasons were?

Don't forget, nothing is too small or insignificant. Small changes are just fine and they might not be many, but keep adding to the list as they occur to you, as you continue to recognise your achievements along the way. You will notice that they will soon become extremely significant as you gather momentum towards your new way of life!

Chapter 3

Reflections / Changes I have noticed since starting this chapter

Daily Checklist towards YOU

Tick these off as you achieve and practice them:

Listed Significant Events and Skills and Attributes I already have	
Listed Skills I want to Develop in the future	
Scored Areas of my Life that need More/Less Attention on the Life Wheel	
Started my Life Action Plan	
Done my Daily Workout	
Done my Daily Visualisation	
Continued to practice 'Me' time	
Written down changes I've already noticed	
Given thanks and gratitude for what I already have and the new knowledge and skills that I am practising	

Summary

Well done you! You are making fantastic progress! You have already achieved so much in such a short space of time in readiness for your continued journey towards your compelling future.

You have realised what wonderful skills and attributes you already have, and have started to make plans to develop new ones. You have also identified the resources that you can call upon to help you on your journey.

Chapter 3

You are practicing your new beliefs and behaviours and are noticing the significant changes that you have brought about. These changes give you the momentum and purpose to continue on your journey to the YOU that you aspire to, and can be.

"

Watch your thoughts for they become words

Watch your words for they become actions

Watch your actions for they become habits

Watch your habits for they become character

Watch your character for it becomes your destiny

Frank Outlaw

"

4

Getting to YOU

This is the chapter where you start revving up your engines. Where you make positive plans for your future and decide just how you are going to get there. You have already identified what areas in your life need more attention, and those that you can now spend less of your valuable time on. Thus, releasing your energy and resources - with my support - will enable you to start to move forward at a rapid pace.

You will now fully define your life's destination, set the scene, choose your supporters and really get going towards the YOU that you want to be!

Goal Setting

We all know the importance of having goals and we set them all the time to help us achieve everything we need to do throughout the day. Without them we would have very little direction and end up becoming frustrated by achieving very little (or nothing at all), using up valuable time and energy in the process!

The good news is that there are only three things you need to get to YOU:

1. A destination - a clear direction to the life you want

2. A Map or SAT NAV - a clear set of values

3. Comfort Breaks – milestones where you can rest along the journey to your destination and check that you are on track

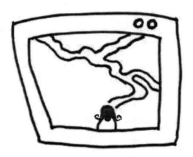

You will always have had goals in your life, no matter how big or small. However, this may be the first time you have ever written them down and made a conscious effort to achieve them in such a structured and time focused way.

Here are a few things to know so that your goals remain at the forefront of your plans.

The key criteria for goals are:

1. **They must be written down.** The physical act of writing down a goal makes it real and tangible. You have no excuse for forgetting about it. As you write, use the word 'will' instead of 'would like to' or 'might'. For

example, 'I will learn to drive'. This statement has power and helps you to 'see' yourself doing it.

2. **Have target dates by which you will achieve your goals.** Your goals must have a realistic deadline and this means that you know when you can celebrate your success. When you are working to a deadline, your sense of urgency increases and achievement will come that much quicker. Remember, small manageable steps help to break down your goals so that you don't feel overwhelmed by them.

3. **Review them daily.** Post sticky notes of your smaller goals in visible places to remind yourself every day of what it is that you intend to do. Put them on your walls, desk, computer monitor, bathroom mirror or refrigerator as a constant reminder. This ensures that you do something towards achieving your goals every single day and they remain at the forefront of your mind.

4. **Have a clearly defined destination.** You already know your destination – *to be* the YOU that you know that you can be. However, don't get so focused on the outcome that you forget to plan all of the steps that are needed along the way.

5. **Having a way of measuring your progress is essential.** By writing out the individual steps towards your goals, and then crossing each one off as you complete them, you'll realise that you are making progress towards your ultimate goal.

6. **Contain a reward for achievement.** Plan rewards as you progress towards your ultimate destination. They may just be small things for achieving your smaller goals but plan to really push the boat out when you achieve the bigger and more significant ones. This will help to motivate you and push you onwards, as well as giving regular achievement highs.

7. **Be set without limits.** Be careful not to set yourself boundaries that may be influenced by your old inner critic or wimp trying to raise its head. Dream big with your new beliefs and behaviours – no wimping out here!

8. **Have a defined support structure.** You already have the inner resources that you need to achieve your goals and you have learned techniques that help you to access these when you need to. In the last chapter, you identified people that can help you on your journey, so ensure that you they are on call for when you need them, even if it's just to give you that extra bit of reassurance if, and when, you need it.

9. **How will you know when you are there?** Only you can answer this one! But be aware, that as you become more self-confident and your behaviours, attitude and outlook change, you might feel that the You, that you aspire to be, appears long before you reach the ultimate long term goal at the end of your journey.

SMART

SMART (or SMARTER) rules will help you to write your own goals in a structured and focused way. SMART is an acronym that helps people to remember something important by using the first letter of a sentence.

So, have a look back at your Life Action Plan(s) in the previous chapter and the goals that you have set for yourself in all of the important areas of your life. Just check that each of them meet the criteria laid out above and below.

If, once you have checked, you find that they need a bit of refining, go ahead and tweak them now. This is an excellent way of checking that your goals are right for you from the outset.

You may find that your shorter term goals change as you progress to achieve your long term ones. That's okay - they are simply a means to an end.

Remember, your journey to YOU is one of self-discovery, and you may find that you steer 'off-road' at some points. Applying the following rules when you define your own goals will ensure that they remain real and achievable for you and keep you on track.

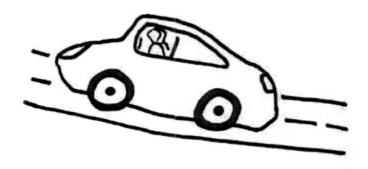

S - Goals must be **Specific** and the more specific the better. State your goal in as exact terms as possible. Your goal must be clear and well defined. Vague or generalised goals are unhelpful because they don't provide sufficient direction for you. Remember, you need goals to show you the way. Think of them as your car headlights showing you the path on your journey. Make it as easy as you can to get where you want to go by defining precisely where you want to end up. Don't be 'woolly' here!

M - Targets should be **Measurable**. That which you measure will be treasured, so think about what will be the measurement of your achievement of your goal. Include precise amounts, dates, etc. in your goals so you can measure your degree of success.

A - Goals should be **Achievable**.

Don't set yourself up to fail here. However, do resist the urge to set goals that are too easy. Accomplishing a goal that you didn't have to work hard for can be anticlimactic at best, and can also make you fear setting future goals that carry a risk of non-achievement. By setting realistic yet challenging goals, you hit the balance you need. These are the types of goals that require you to 'raise the bar' and they bring you the greatest personal satisfaction.

R - Goals must be **Realistic**.

Unrealistic goals will lead to discouragement. Remember: small, easy steps. Don't set yourself up to fail at the first hurdle. Goals should be relevant to the direction you want your life to take. By keeping goals in line with this direction, you'll develop the focus you need to get ahead and do what you want. Set widely scattered and inconsistent goals and you'll fritter your time – and your life – away.

T – **Targets**. Targets should be time based.

Decide your timetable for completion, and stick to it. Make sure you include some 'quick wins' too.

E - Goals should be **Exciting** and you should have **Enthusiasm**. Exciting goals will be met far sooner than boring, bland ones that don't excite and energise you towards them.

R - Goals should be **Recorded** and **Rewarded**, in a place where you can look at them every day. That means writing them down, looking at them every day and making steps towards them every day, so that they become so real that you can't stop yourself from moving towards them. Do something towards your goal every single day and see the rewards, both short and long term!

You've done some really good work and have started to create your new future towards the real YOU now.

However, remember to practice the techniques and exercises from the previous chapters to motivate and energise you to continue your momentum. You have all of the resources that you need to achieve your goals inside of you.

Remember your poster sized collage of all the parts that will make YOU? You created it in chapter one, and now is the time to add your goals to it. You might like to print off the goals you will be working on immediately and stick them to your poster, so that you see them every day, so that you feel motivated and reminded to take small actions every day towards your bigger goals. Remember to post your smaller goals on sticky notes in prominent places so that you complete one every day!

You may have found the previous task hard work, but you will be rewarded many times over for laying the groundwork to help your make your dreams real.

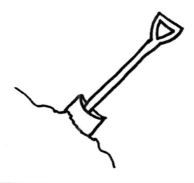

Daily Workout

Your Ideal Week

1. Relax (close your eyes if it helps) and take a few deep breaths. Now vividly imagine what your life will look like as you are living as YOU. What will you see? What will you hear? How do you speak? How does it feel? As you do this, really imagine living your life as YOU, in as much detail as you possibly can. Create a rich inner experience as if you are already living your future YOU now.

2. Next use everything you have learned about what you want, what really matters to you, and what your ultimate goal is - and pour them all into your ideal week.

3. How does your week begin? On what day does it start? Imagine the kind of people you have around you, the places that you go, the things you have around you. How good do you feel? Where do you go each day? How do you spend your time? Who do you see? What are the things that let you know that you have achieved everything that you set out to do?

4. Continue to go through your ideal week, day by day, until you can imagine every detail really vividly. Just indulge yourself, take your time and enjoy the positive feelings the exercise gives you.

And now for your daily visualisation to practice...

Daily Visualisation

Creating Your Future Vision Today

Relax and close your eyes if it helps you.

1. Imagine you are flying through time and space to a year in the future and you have had the best year of your life.

   What has happened to your job/career, your relationships, your health, your money/wealth? Wellbeing? What new behaviours and state of mind are you practicing? Who are you with? Who are you becoming? What do you look like? Sound like? How do you feel?

   Which of your short term goals have already been achieved? Which ones became less important as you progressed? Which longer term goals are already moving along nicely?

   What is it like to live the life you want every day? How have your values and beliefs changed? Which ones are now more important to you? Which ones seem less so, or have been left on the wayside of your journey towards your goals and the life you want to have?

2. Now, imagine an ideal picture or short movie that represents everything that you want to happen in your positive future. Make sure you can see yourself in the picture of your future looking totally confident, positive and extremely happy.

   Create you ideal picture or short movie now. Where are you? Who is with you? What makes your life so much richer and pleasurable? What are you satisfied most with?

3. Put your picture or movie onto your timeline one year into your future. Make sure it's really big, bold, bright and colourful.

4. Next, fill in the gaps between then and now.

   - Make a slightly smaller picture or movie 'still' and place it a few months before the big picture of what needs to happen before that.

   - Make an even smaller picture or movie 'still' and place it a few months before that picture of what needs to happen before that.

   - Make an even smaller picture or movie 'still' and place it a few months before that picture of what needs to happen before that.

   You should now have a string of pictures or movie 'stills' that connect the present with your positive future, your bright future. The pictures should get progressively bigger with better and better things happening in them.

5. Look at your picture 'string' and let your unconscious mind lock in the Sat Nav route map to your new life over the next year.

6. Now float up and out of your body and into each picture. Take your time to fully experience each step you will be taking on this journey towards the YOU that you know that you can be.

7. When you get to the big picture of your ideal future, really immerse yourself in it and enjoy the experience. What will it be like to have everything you want?

8. Finally, come back to now, and look out once again to your future timeline. You can feel confident that you have

created a Sat Nav route for your unconscious mind to use as a guide for bringing your ideal future into reality.

You can repeat both of the above exercises as often as you like, either by reading it through by or by listening to the weblink at *www.the-change-coach.co.uk*, and each time you do you will move closer towards the future YOU that you know you can be.

Me Time

You have done a lot of good work on your future during this chapter and I hope you took time, and are still taking regular time out, to recharge your energy supplies. This time to yourself should now be a regular part of your daily routine – not a guilty pleasure.

Don't become complacent in trying out new experiences and pushing your boundaries and getting out of your comfort zone; you are still on your journey and should remain open to new ideas, as many of these experiences will enhance and enrich your journey.

The Daily Workout in this chapter can be used regularly during 'Me' time and is a good exercise to do whilst listening to gentle music as it will help to reinforce your vision of your future and explore other possibilities that may just pop into your mind, as you allow yourself to relax and daydream your future into reality.

Time to Reflect and to Celebrate your progress

Reflections / Changes I have noticed already

Daily Checklist towards YOU

Tick these off as you achieve and practice them

Revisited my Life Action Plan and tweaked each important area, applying the Key Criteria for Goals and SMARTER	
Done my Daily Workout	
Done my Daily Visualisation	
Continued to practice 'Me' time	
Written down changes I've already noticed	
Given thanks and gratitude for what I already have and the new knowledge and skills that I am practising	

Summary

Phew – time to take a breather from what must have seemed like an extremely thorough process, but you have made some important adjustments to your Life Action Plan(s) and completed a systematic review of your goals that will navigate you to complete your journey to YOU.

You have clearly identified what you need to do, what resources you need, and when you need to have achieved certain tasks by.

You have imagined your future vividly in pictures with specific content and dates to keep you focussed and are practising taking precious 'Me' time, which will provide you with the energy and motivation you need, as you take the actions required to achieve those smaller goals along your journey, towards your now extremely vivid future.

Chapter 4

The good news is that the fun starts now! A place where you can start experimenting with ideas and thoughts to sharpen your picture of the ideal You that you can be!

Onwards!

"

Setting goals is the first step in turning the invisible into the visible

Tony Robbins

"

5

Creating the Real YOU

Chapter 5 takes a positive look and review of your current self-image. It provides ways to turn down the volume, once and for all, on your critical self. It gives you several techniques to practice, to further increase your confidence, to continue to transform yourself in readiness to embrace the new era of your life that you are travelling towards.

We are going to work at channelling all of that energy - that may be currently directed at holding on to that old negative self-image - into a newly polished self-image or a new sparkling reality with positive reinforcements of your improved self-image.

What is Self-Image?

Your self-image is the way you see yourself in your mind. These are the internal pictures, sounds and feelings of ourselves that we recognise as 'us'. Self-image may be how you see yourself physically, or your opinion of *who* and *what* you are (which is normally called self-concept). It is important as it affects your self-esteem and confidence. Self-image is really powerful because your behaviour will almost never swerve away from this internal picture. Your mind behaves consistently with the kind of person that you *think* you are.

Many people are not aware of their own self-image until they really look! We are usually preoccupied with the images that bombard us in the media every day and of the people around us, rarely taking time to examine our own.

Self-image includes:

- What you think you look like
- How you see your personality
- What kind of person you think you are
- What you believe others think of you
- How much you like yourself or think others like you
- The status you feel you have
- How you think you should dress and behave according to your age

What does self-image have to do with self-esteem?

Self-esteem is how you *feel* about yourself. Image is about how you *see* yourself and how you believe others see you. They are closely connected because if you have a poor self-image or opinion of yourself - your self-esteem will be low.

Image is to do with perception. How you see yourself is vital because this will affect your behaviour, your thinking, and how you relate to others. People respond to you either positively or negatively according to how confident you are. Your confidence in relationships depends on the image you have of yourself.

How *you* see yourself is often different from how *others* view you. Your view of yourself is shaped by your unique thoughts and beliefs and you will have a distorted view. You will see yourself in a positive or negative way according to your level of self-esteem. You may have a negative view of yourself and, if so, you are probably highly critical of yourself. We all know people, and we may be guilty of this ourselves, that think they are either too fat, too thin, too shy, too old, or too 'something else'.

The problem is that anyone who really believes, and consistently tells themselves (and others) that they are too fat, too thin, or too whatever creates a self-fulfilling prophecy. They will unconsciously sabotage any attempts to appear attractive. Because they don't project themselves at their best, people will inevitably find them less attractive and so the cycle continues.

This is a learned behaviour that becomes a habit. You are projecting your own opinion of yourself to others. Who are they to challenge this if you don't challenge it yourself?

Our own self-image has been formed over many years and has been affected by many events and influences in our lives, many since childhood. Many of our earliest messages from childhood were positive and encouraging, but many were often outweighed by criticism from our parents, teachers, and other role models. Unfortunately comments such as 'you clumsy/silly/big/naughty girl' are the ones that really stick in our minds and go on to form our own opinion and self-image and self-esteem over the years into adulthood.

We tend to remember the negative comments and experiences much more than the positive ones, and the hurt feelings stay with us, as they have the biggest impact.

Chapter 5

It doesn't help that many cultures quash any successes that we achieve and even appear fearful of celebrating achievements. We have all heard it said as a child: "nobody likes a show-off". No wonder we form negative self-images of ourselves, resulting in low self-esteem, as we grow into adults!

Try the following exercise to help you to recognise whether you are still holding on to any negative comments that have gone on to form negative habits about yourself, into adulthood.

Daily Workout

1. Revisit a couple of those negative memories that you had as a child, teenager or young adult, where someone made a comment that really hurt, that you have carried with you to this day.

2. Imagine the scene. See what you saw, hear what was said and the tone. Feel what you felt.

3. Play the scene as a movie in your mind but *not* through the eyes of the child/teenager/adult that you were.

    Play the movie through your own eyes as an adult, standing nearby and observing what happened from a distance. Play the movie forward in black and white and then run it backwards in colour. Do this a couple of times, running it faster and faster each time, backwards and forwards until you can't get the feeling, or the memory seems distant.

4. Where's the emotion, as you view the scene as an adult with your grown up knowledge? Is it there, or is it less intense? What else do you notice? That they were just

kids? And isn't that just what kids do? Kids can sometimes be spiteful and bullies. Most times, kids don't know any better.

I'm sure the same people would be mortified if they knew that that the comments they made had such an impact on you, and shaped you into the adult that you are today.

5. If you can still access the memory, keep looking at the scene and notice how you as a child/teenager/young adult handled it. Then go over it, and give that younger you an invisible hug and whisper some words of wisdom that you wouldn't have known then, but do now as an adult.

6. If the hurtful comments were made by an adult, such as a teacher or parent - do the same exercise and ask yourself, "what was their intention?" Was it to protect you, advise you, help you? They may have had a particular way of saying things, and sometimes (with hindsight) you realise it was 'just their way'. They may have not known any different.

    If you think the comments were made just to be spiteful or vindictive, then they are just playground bullies who have grown up to be bullies as adults. It does happen! However, it does help to take the emotion out of the memory and apply your adult knowledge to it. Learn from the experience with your new positive outlook.

    Don't allow yourself to remain at 'effect'. You are in control here. Don't allow them to continue to hurt you, they probably don't even remember saying it, so don't waste any more of your time and energy dwelling on it – move on and let go.

Repeat this exercise each time you think of a negative experience in your past that you think is still having an impact on your behaviour or how you see yourself today. Alternatively, listen to the weblink at *www.the-change-coach.co.uk*

Now that you have taken out some of the emotion from the negative experiences from childhood and learned from them, you can now move on and look at ways to improve your self-image and self-esteem. If you can change your thinking, your behaviour will invariably follow.

Why does looking after your Self-image and Self-esteem matter?

Your opinion of yourself, what you think of your own 'worth', really does make a difference to your life. If you *mistakenly* value yourself too low, many things can go wrong. You may:

- blame yourself for things that aren't your fault
- underestimate your own abilities
- expect things to go wrong for you

But when you have an appropriate, balanced view of yourself, you can:

- be much fairer on yourself
- be more objective about your strong points
- have more confidence in your abilities
- feel calmer when you think about yourself and your future
- think more positively about life generally

So, rather than going flat out for *high* self-esteem, the best way forward is to work on building it to a *healthy level* that will help you get more out of life and feel more comfortable with yourself. Remember, small, manageable steps...

Now let's have a look at how you perceive your self-image at the moment, before describing the self-image that you *want* to have (think of your role model if you have one) in the future, when you reach your long term goal. Complete the columns below.

My Self-image of Myself

Now	Future

If you prefer, you can cut out pictures from magazines or simply draw pictures that represent the self-image that you are developing for the future YOU, and paste or add them to your goal poster. Then, you can see them every day and keep working towards making them a reality.

Now, take a look back on your responses to some of the exercises in the previous chapters, particularly at your current skills and attributes and those that you wanted to develop.

With these in mind, look back at what you have written in the table above. Can you think of anything else that you would like to add?

Mirror, Mirror....

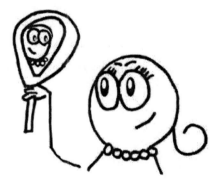

So, we know that your self-image is the one that you show to the world, but is it the true image of yourself that you are projecting?

When you look at yourself in the mirror every morning, you never think to question whether the person you see is actually *you*. We accept the image in the mirror as the one we see every day. We recognise the woman in the mirror in front of us – it's the one who went to bed last night and woke up this morning, maybe a bit more dishevelled, but the same!

But do we really stop and see the real you, or the one you want to be?

You feel familiar - at home with your own unique self-image. This familiarity is comfortable in itself - we know it and live with it every day, it's easy not to challenge it, isn't it? You may be surprised to learn that many extremely confident and successful people are quite shy and insecure underneath the surface, but it's their self-image that tells the world that 'I have it all' that we notice most. They cultivate this image and we are convinced it's true. Many famous and successful people today have stylists who create an image for them which they continually promote to the outside world.

This is pretty powerful stuff that you can start to learn and use to your own advantage.

So, we know that image and appearance are important, as it influences the opinions and impressions of those around us. We don't have a professional stylist on hand to dish out expensive advice, so we will take a systematic look at your personal appearance and image projection as it is now. Then you can decide whether it needs changing or not, to fit the future YOU that you are moving towards.

I did say at the beginning of your journey that I will encourage and challenge you to step outside your comfort zone. Now, I'm telling you to jump right out of it. You are so much more confident now and this is just another milestone in your journey. So, don't be afraid, as I will be here to guide you when things get tough.

Let's now take a positive but critical audit of your self-image and personal appearance and check whether it needs refining, to help increase your self-esteem and project the image of the YOU that you want.

As the old saying goes: "if you always do what you always did, then you will always get what you always got" and that's *not* why you began your journey to YOU is it?

Body Image

Now, I want you to take a critical, but positive look at your physical appearance. The image of yourself that you carry with you and are currently projecting to the rest of the world.

This may not be something you do too often, or are comfortable with, but it's just you by yourself, and we are going to conduct a bit of an MOT check on your attributes and learn to celebrate the good bits and stop dismissing any flaws that you feel you have. This is a positive exercise!

Overlook the flaws. It might sound silly, but just smiling at yourself in the mirror helps you to look at yourself in a positive light.

Take a long look in a full length mirror if you have one.

Now we are going to conduct a top-to-toe audit of yourself to enable you to judge for yourself whether anything needs improving or not. Be honest with yourself, but watch out that you don't become over critical – quell that inner critic!

You may find that once you have completed this task that your current self-image does not require much work and just needs some updating. Alternatively, you might decide that it needs a good old clear out and embrace the new ideas that the new, confident you is itching to try out.

Top to Toe Image Audit

Ask yourself the following questions and try to be as objective as possible. Tackle the task as if you have just met yourself for the first time, and as you progress, mark the table below with a cross or a tick, depending on what areas you decide need attention. You might like to add notes as you progress, so note down your immediate thoughts. Don't dwell too deeply.

1. **What are the things about my body that I'm most proud of**, or I like best?

2. **What's my posture like?** How do I stand? Confident or slouched or in between?

3. **What habits do I have that others notice?** Nail biting, clearing my throat, playing with my ear lobes, etc.

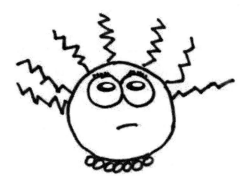

4. **Hair** – do I use my hair to hide my face? Does the style and colour suit my face and age? Does the style suit the thickness, thinness, texture or condition of it? How long have I had it in the current style? How much maintenance does it need?

5. **Face** – what condition is my skin in? Do I need to update my skincare regime? Check for colour, pigmentation, broken veins, blemishes, skin conditions, lines, wrinkles, warts, moles. Does the presence of any of these affect my confidence when I meet people for the first time?

6. **Make-up** – do I wear it? Should I wear it? Is what I wear suitable for the image I want to portray? Is it outdated? Does my foundation still match my skin tone? Do the colours complement me?

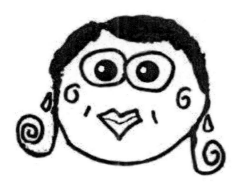

7. **Eye Brows** – are they plucked? Over plucked? Do they shape my face? Are they the correct thickness and colour for me?

8. **Eyes**. Really notice the colour. If I wear glasses, do they suit my face and colouring? Have I considered contact lenses or laser surgery if they are a high prescription and impede my lifestyle? Do I make the most of them? Do I draw attention to them?

9. **Lips** – are they moist and well defined?

10. **Mouth** – are my teeth regular and white? Do I see the dentist regularly? Have I got fresh breath? Do I smile readily or I am I embarrassed about my teeth?

11. **Facial Hair** – do I have excess hair on my face? If so, do I know what options I have to remove it?

12. **Piercings** – are people that I meet for the first time drawn to them first, and form an opinion of me? Are they appropriate for the new image I want to project to other people?

13. **Neck** – do I hold my chin up? Does it need toning?

14. **Décolletage** – is it sun damaged? Lined?

15. **Bust** – am I wearing the correct size bra and cup size? Is my lingerie faded or outdated?

16. **Weight/muscle tone/fitness** – are there areas that require toning?

17. **Tattoos** - are they visible? Are they appropriate for the new image I want to project to other people?

18. **Finger/toe nails** – are they healthy? Manicured?

19. **Clothes** – is my current style suitable for my size, height and age? Are they well maintained? Am I hanging on to clothes that I had years ago in a range of different sizes?

20. **Shoes** - is my current style and range suitable for my size, height and age?

21. **Accessories** – do I have any? Do they complement me and my clothes or do they draw attention from me?

Top-to-Toe Checklist

Things I like best about my body/self:

Posture:

Habits:

Hair:

Face:

Make up:

Eye Brows:

Eyes:

Lips:

Mouth:

Facial Hair:

Piercings:

Neck:

Décolletage:

Bust:

Weight/muscle tone/fitness:

Tattoos:

Finger/toe nails:

Clothes:

Shoes:

Accessories:

How did you do? Don't forget, this is your opinion and you are your strongest critic! You might want to ask yourself whether your old inner critic or wimp was sitting on your shoulder whilst you conducted your audit.

If you feel that this is the case, you could ask a trusted friend to give an objective opinion and check if they agree with your own findings. Be careful who you choose, it needs to be someone who does not have a hidden agenda, someone who could sabotage the great progress you have made so far.

Choose someone, who is open to new ideas, is creative and wants the very best for you.

If their trusted opinion is pretty close to your own findings, good, you managed to remain objective throughout your audit, so well done!

If this wasn't the case, check that those old limiting beliefs are not trying to creep back into your consciousness. Put on your ring of energy and motivation and repeat some of your daily visualisations, to help you to get back into your confident zone.

With this new additional knowledge, you might like to review your top-to-toe audit for specific actions that you might decide to take, and add them to your goals. Begin to explore some options and add them to the significant changes that you have already made. Now the fun starts. So get out those sticky notes again and start writing!

Here are some specific ideas that you might consider if you get stuck for inspiration. But *you* are your best guide, be creative and really go for it:

Don't overlook the things that you like best about yourself. Exploit and celebrate them. Ask yourself how you can promote them to your best advantage.

- **Posture** – standing tall and straight with your shoulders back adds inches to you and immediately says that you are confident. Practice walking confidently and with ease, if this is not already second nature to you.

- **Personal habits** – whether this is nail biting, smoking or just nervous laughter, think about the impact it is having on your self-image and your confidence. What are the options available to you to get rid of it, if you choose to? You may find some of them just disappear as your confidence and self-esteem increase, but consider your options from practicing the techniques in this workbook to hypnotherapy and relaxation. The options are varied so look around to what suits your budget.

- **Hair** – have you used the same hairdresser for years? Have you used your hair to hide your face? Are you brave enough to try something new to fit with your new image? There are lots of model nights around or try your local college where you can evaluate new styles and colours that are inexpensive. Someone new will also give you an objective opinion on what suits your face and lifestyle.
  Some hairdressers even have computer software where they take a photograph of you and superimpose different hairstyles and colours onscreen so you can choose which ones suit you.

- **Face** – this is the face that you show to the world and were born with (for most of us anyway), so celebrate its uniqueness. Notice what expression you choose to wear on it though. Is it friendly and open? Do you tend to frown a lot? This is something that you can change if you want to. Just practice it often and notice the responses you get!

- **Make up** – now this is something you can have fun with as your naked face is indeed a blank canvass. If you have never really bothered with make-up or are unsure how to apply it or what suits you, have fun experimenting. Go along to a large department store's make-up counters, early in the day when they are less busy. Take a friend if you need to, make a day of it. Ask for a free make-up lesson or some trial products for you to try at home. You don't have to buy anything and, again as they don't know you, they will provide you with professional, impartial advice on what suits you best.

- **Eye Brows** – these help to frame our face and tend to get neglected. There are now eye brow stencils that you can practice shading in with brow pencils or alternatively try a brow bar or beauty salon in your high street that can advise you on shape, thickness and colour. If you have over plucked them and they are now thin with no regrowth, you can even have them tattooed on. This applies to your eye and lip liner too and is much longer lasting, if expensive, but may be an option for you.

- **Eyes** – these are allegedly the windows to your soul, so make the most of them. If you wear glasses and think that they need an update there are so many different styles these days. Book an appointment or just browse in a store that has a wide variety to choose from. There are usually good deals where you receive a pair free, so it's good to shop around. Have you considered wearing contact lenses to fit with your new self-image and lifestyle? They are so much easier to wear and don't require the care that previous ones used to. Most opticians offer a monthly payment plan, so they are more affordable. You can even try different coloured ones for an alternative look.

Your experiments with make-up may have given you new skills with which to make the most of your eyes. What about false eyelashes for some special occasions, or even eye lash extensions if yours aren't particularly long or thick? There are also 24 hour eyeliners available or, just as you can with your eyebrows, eyeliner tattoos are available for a longer term alternative.

- **Lips** – balms, lipstick and gloss can be used to enhance your lips. Lip liner will provide you with a defined lip line if yours are a bit indistinct.

- **Mouth** – your smile instantly brightens up your face and mood. Do you have a dentist? Do you visit them regularly? If not, are you afraid to? As well as checking your teeth for plaque or decay, your dentist also checks for gum disease and other potential oral problems, so it's an investment against future health issues in this area.

  If you are embarrassed about your teeth, there are options available to have them whitened or straightened if necessary, so your dentist can advise and provide you with a free quote and explanation of the work needed, with payment plans too.

- **Facial Hair** – some cultures naturally have noticeable fine facial hair. However, if you have a problem with excessive facial hair this may be a sign of polycystic ovaries, which encourages hair growth; testosterone can cause it; or you may have a genetic disposition towards it, so see you GP to check it out.

  If you have excessive facial hair - coarse hairs have appeared as you have gotten older, there are many treatment options that you can consider if you are conscious or embarrassed about it. These range from threading, waxing, bleaching to laser, Intense Pulsed Light (IPL) to electronic gadgets that you can use at home. If you are considering any of these routes, ask for special offers at your local salon (check they are registered practitioners) or try your local college.

- **Piercings** – this is something you chose to have, so if they no longer meet your needs you can remove them. If they do, leave them where they are. They are all part of your individuality. Just check that they are still part of the self-image that you are developing further for your future.

- **Neck** – Do you hold your head high? Or do you constantly look at the floor as you walk? As with your posture, looking straight ahead and making eye contact with people tells the world that you are a confident woman. You also see and notice so much more!

- **Décolletage** – This is the area below your neck, at the top of your chest between your shoulders. If this area is sun damaged or lined, you might wish to protect it by disguising it with pretty scarves or necklaces to draw attention away from it. If not, use SPF and flaunt it, as appropriate.

- **Bust** – Are you wearing the correct bra and cup size? A well fitted bra can make all the difference to how comfortable you feel and the way your clothes hang on you. Many high street stores offer a bra fitting service that is professional and unobtrusive. Pretty underwear is a confidence booster in itself, so go and experiment! More importantly, don't forget to check your breasts regularly for any changes or lumps.

- **Weight/muscle tone/fitness** – is your weight or your level of fitness affecting your confidence? You are your most precious asset and being in control of both of these areas will provide you with added energy and vigour to continue to move closer to your goals of being the YOU that you are well on the road to being. Even small healthy changes to your eating habits and by starting with short walks and doing something differently, like taking the stairs instead of the lift, will start the momentum you may need to increase your energy output.

- **Tattoos** – once again, this is something you chose to have. It may have been to remember something by, or as a marker of a significant event in your life. However, if they no longer meet the needs of your new, future self, they are more painful, costly and difficult to remove than piercings. They are all part of your individuality. You may even be contemplating having one done to celebrate your progress so far! Just consider the longer term impact of where it's positioned!

- **Finger/Toe Nails** – well manicured nails will be noticed by others and do create an impression of good personal grooming. If you bite your fingernails there are products on the market to help you stop doing this or you could consider visiting a nail salon and having gel or acrylic nails to help you to break the habit.

- **Clothes** – Clothes are the easiest way to create an impression and update your self-image and this is where you can have the most fun in trying out new ideas. The good news is that this exercise doesn't have to be expensive. You will need to have an idea on the changes that you want to make to update or improve your self-image first.

You could start by getting everything out of your wardrobe and separating the clothes that you already have, with the image that you want to project to others. Be strict with yourself and bag up everything that doesn't match these criteria for the charity shop. You might like to pull in your trusted friend (TF) again here to keep you disciplined! Be ruthless and include the outfits that no longer fit you, or those that you have kept for years just because you had spent a lot of money on them. They won't be of use to you in the future.

With what's left, mix and match them into different outfits that you perhaps hadn't considered before, and try each of them on. Take your time, put some music on and make an evening out of it – have fun! Next, make a list of what you still need to complete your wardrobe to help you to create your new image. If you still need some inspiration, book an appointment with a personal shopper at a large department store, and take your TF with you. These are not intimidating and you will not be expected to buy anything unless you choose to. Ensure that you provide your personal shopper with an exact brief of what you are looking for. For example, you could say that you are recreating yourself (which is true) and give her an idea of what you are after. She will select items that she thinks meets your criteria and bring a selection to your changing room, which is usually larger and more private than the other fitting rooms on the shop floor.

Before you go, ensure you wear well fitted underwear

(you could have your bra fitted at the same time), as well fitted foundation garments make all the difference to how clothes hang on you. Check that your bra doesn't cut into you and that you don't have a visible panty line – make full use of the mirrors and lighting there.

Don't be tempted to buy everything that's suggested to you, you can just go away and think about it. There is no need to feel pressured into buying. This is more of a learning experience than a shopping trip. Take a notebook with you and make a note of what styles, colours, sizes and lengths suit and flatter you most.

- **Shoes** – the same goes for shoes, sandals and boots. Throw out any that are uncomfortable and try on lots of different styles and heights. Notice what flatters you the most and try to stick with it. Sometimes it's better to buy a more expensive brand that are comfortable and which flatter you rather than buying lots of different cheaper pairs that you won't wear.

- **Accessories** – this is where you can be at your most creative. Bright, bold scarves, necklaces, bracelets and bags can make a difference to any outfit and change the look of one at very little expense. Once you have decided on the look that you want to achieve, and what will become your 'signature' style, wear the outfits when you are next out shopping. Experiment with different looks that you can use with several different outfits and add accessories as they catch your eye. Charity shops and car boot sales are a great way to try things out at minimal cost.

Above all, try something new and play with ideas. You can dismiss most or even all of the above, but the thing is that you gave it a go, learned from the experience and whatever you decided is what's best for you.

Keep asking for feedback from positive trusted people in your life and take time to plan what you are going to wear for every occasion, even if it's just to walk to the shops. You have invested a lot of time, effort and energy in cultivating your self-image, so take the time to continually develop and flaunt it – because you're worth every minute of it.

First Impressions

It's said that it takes 3 seconds for someone to establish an impression of someone when meeting them for the first time. When it comes to making the first, and lasting impression, body language as well as appearance speaks much louder than words.

Now that you have revitalised your individual style, use your body language and posture to project appropriate confidence and self-assurance. Stand tall, smile, make eye contact, and greet people warmly, as if you are genuinely pleased to see them. Make them feel special. All of this will help you project self-assurance and encourage you to feel better at ease, as your confidence and self-esteem increase.

First Meetings

Almost everyone gets a little nervous when meeting someone for the first time, which can lead to nervous habits or sweaty palms. Prepare for a first meeting by practising some of the exercises in the previous chapters, and imagining it going smoothly, just the way that you want it. This will take most of the stress out of the event.

By being aware of your nervous habits, you can try to keep them in check. And controlling a nervous habit or a nervous laugh will give you confidence. Relaxation practiced during 'Me' time can help with this.

If nerves get the better of you, take a few moments and breathe deeply. Try to remember a time when you handled a tough situation and came out triumphantly. Use what you learned from these experiences to be confident in the current situation.

Of course, physical appearance matters. The person you are meeting for the first time does not know you, and your appearance is usually the first clue he or she has to go on. The more comfortable you are with yourself, and with what you are wearing, will go a long way in helping you to create a positive impression.

They say a picture is worth a thousand words, and so the 'picture' you first present says much about you to the person you are meeting. Is your appearance saying the right things that you want to convey to help create the right first impression?

Individuality

The good news is that you can usually create a good impression without losing your individuality. Yes, to make a good first impression you do need to 'fit in' to some degree. But it all goes back to being appropriate for the situation.

Although occasions are much less formal these days, always check out what's required dress wise, to prevent any embarrassing mistakes. Wear an outfit for the occasion. If in a business setting, wear appropriate business clothes. If it's at a formal evening social event, wear appropriate evening dress. And express your individuality appropriately within that context.

Chapter 5

A Winning Smile!

There's nothing like a smile to create a good first impression. A warm and confident smile will put both you and the other person at ease. Someone who smiles a lot can appear much more approachable and at ease with themselves, even if they aren't underneath!

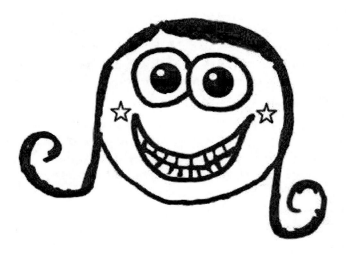

Be Positive

Your attitude shows through in everything you do. Project your positive attitude, even in the face of extreme nervousness or anxiety. And smile your confident smile.

Daily Visualisation

Read the following exercise though a few times before you begin, so that you know what to do. You might want to light some scented candles and play soft music too.

Bringing it all Together

1. Sit yourself in a comfortable chair or lie down if you prefer

2. Close your eyes and take a few deep breaths and just become aware of your breathing for a few moments. As you relax, imagine a wave of warm relaxation, gently beginning to flow downwards through your body. As the wave progresses, relax each muscle until it reaches your toes.

3. Then start to remember how you felt when you began your journey towards the YOU that you want to be, and nearly are. Remember the thoughts that you had. Remember the commitment that you made to yourself.

4. Remember the daily workouts and visualisations that you have practiced. What are you favourites? What have made the most difference to your behaviour and thoughts?

5. Remember letting go of the old limiting beliefs? The old inner critic? How good it feels to have let go...

6. Feel how good it is to have made so much progress to the YOU that you know you can be. To have ticked off so many of those smaller goals to move

you to your ultimate one.

7.   Look out to the future and see the confident YOU,
     with abundant self-belief and esteem. Look at how
     she walks, speaks, feels. Notice her style. What she's
     wearing. That's right.

Repeat this exercise whenever you like. Keep the vision and
feelings real for you. Alternatively, listen to the weblink at
www.the-change-coach.co.uk

Me Time Maximisers

Your 'Me' time should be an indulgent habit by now, with
you being able to experience some peace and serenity by
yourself, every single day. But what about a few 'Me'
maximisers as a special treat to yourself every now and again?
Especially as you reach a major milestone on your journey
towards YOU.

These treats may take some time to plan, but the anticipation
will make them all the more rewarding and enjoyable. They
don't have to be expensive, and you might like to consider
some of the following, or let your imagination go wild:

*   **A day of rest and recuperation** (or half if you can't
    manage a full day!) - During the week work and other
    commitments tend to take over your time and energy,
    so why not make your home into a haven and plan a
    day spa there? Get everything you will need in
    advance, so you don't have to leave the house. Have a
    lie in, take a leisurely bath with your favourite bubbles
    or oils, scented candles and start to give yourself the
    top to toe treatment and enjoy!

- **Take a hike** - As well as helping to lower blood pressure and lose body fat, walking outdoors is associated with mental well-being. It also helps self-esteem and some symptoms of depression. It doesn't have to be a major trek, maybe just around your local park or area. Borrow a dog if you don't have one yourself. Just get out there and explore. Take time to look around you and notice things you may have not noticed before. Slow down, look up, notice the trees, the buildings, anything new to you.

- **Meet up with positive friends or loved ones** - Although this is 'Me' time, sometimes you receive an energy boost from other positive people that will give you food for thought to reflect on next time you are alone. Take time to enjoy the experience. Ask them questions about themselves that you don't already know. Don't rush it, give yourself plenty of time to arrive at the meeting point and don't arrange anything immediately afterwards, so that you don't need to rush off.

- **Do Something Different by Yourself** - Is there something that you wish that you had tried or visited but just haven't made the time previously to do? It could be anything from learning to make Dim Sum to visiting a specialist travel agent to plan a long haul trip. Be adventurous!

Chapter 5

Reflections / Changes I have noticed

Daily Checklist towards YOU

Tick these off as you achieve and practice them

Listed Current and Future Self-image	
Top-to-Toe Checklist	
Done my Daily Workout	
Done my Daily Visualisation	
Planned and Practiced 'Me' time maximisers	
Written down changes I've noticed since starting this chapter	
Ticked off progress I have made towards my goals	

Summary

You have experienced several challenges in this chapter and have had to jump right outside of your comfort zone. You have revisited some negative memories in your Daily Workout and should have removed some of the emotions attached to those memories, to help you learn and to move on from them.

You have examined your self-image and conducted an objective top-to-toe audit on it, to help you identify what parts of your self-image need attention, those that you can flaunt, and those parts that are potentially hindering your progress, as you move ever closer towards the YOU that you aspire to be.

Chapter 5

You have had some fun experimenting with new ideas, including maximising some of your 'Me' time.

I expect your reflections for this chapter to be fairly lengthy, but with lots of new learning and knowledge included in them. You have already achieved so much now, I'm so proud of you. You are nearly there, so let's continue to the final stages of your journey with your new found knowledge, enthusiasm and momentum – come on!

In pursuit of learning, something is acquired.

In pursuit of freedom, every day something is dropped

Lao Tsu

"

6

Keeping it Real – YOU Maintenance

Well, here you are – nearly at the end of your journey of self-discovery to finding your way back to YOU.

At the start of your journey, you made a commitment to yourself to fulfil your true potential and you are now so very nearly there. You have maintained your self-belief, and invested your time and energy over several months to get to where you are today.

There have been challenges along the way and, I hope, lots of fun and several 'wow' moments, when you realised the impact that taking even those small steps in your development towards YOU have already made.

This final chapter will encourage you to reflect on the positive changes you have made to your life, and to learn from what has challenged you. It will provide you with further techniques that will ensure that you continue to move towards your new fulfilling future. The future you set out to achieve at the beginning of our time together.

Keeping it Real – What Next?

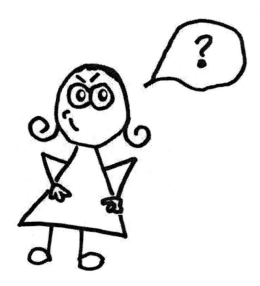

Many of us strive to achieve something significant at different times in our lives. Be it passing an important exam, learning to drive, or securing our first home.

We could be focused on a particular date or achieving a certain amount of money or all manner of material things. We work hard and make sacrifices to achieve these goals and bask in the satisfaction when we have achieved them for a while - until the memory or achievement no longer has such an impact as we move on to the next challenge. Or we are just satisfied that achieving a particular goal was so huge that the satisfaction lasts for a significant time.

However we have all known, or heard of, people who have achieved great success and appear to have everything they aspired for and worked hard for, only to appear to lose their sense of purpose and direction once they have achieved it.

You have made significant changes to your behaviour and progress towards achieving your goals already, so be alert to complacency and procrastination, particularly when you have achieved your more significant goals.

You may find that once you have achieved your most significant goals that your future ones are not as challenging to get to as the ones you have already arrived at. However, you have done the difficult part and have learned new behaviours that got you to where you are now.

Looking after the positive changes you have made is a major part of helping you to stay focussed and for the maintenance of YOU. You can nurture your new beliefs and behaviours every day. It's a bit like watering a flower to keep it thriving. The more care you take of yourself, generally and more specifically, by practising your new ways of thinking and being, the more you reduce the chances of returning to your previous self.

Keeping the Weeds Out of your Future

Try thinking of your life as a beautiful garden. Unhealthy ways of thinking and your old ways of behaving, including influences from Moodhoovers and Energy Vampires around you, are the weeds in your garden. While the beautiful flowers in your garden are your new ways of behaviour, such as being confident, motivated, with focused energy and increased self-esteem - your new ways of living.

No garden is ever weed-free and these blighters will constantly try to creep in, unnoticed amongst your flowers. You need to continuously water and feed your flowers, giving them plenty of exposure to sunlight, picking out any weeds as soon as they appear, to keep your garden healthy. You may need to use some weed killer on those weeds now and again, so keep practicing your Daily Workouts and Visualisations, or anything else you have stored in your personal resource bank to blitz them as soon as they appear! Never ignore them - be vigilant in your garden.

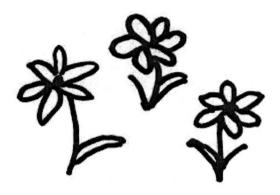

If at any time you find your old inner critic or wimp trying to make a comeback, look back on what motivated you and moved you forward during your journey. You already know what motivates you and provides you with the energy and enthusiasm to get where you want to be. Every good gardener talks to their flowers, so, if it helps to quell that inner critic or wimp, give those weeds a good old talking to!

In turn, recognise when you start to 'coast' along. Get moving, get busy, get focused on your compelling future.

Repeat some of the techniques to get you re-energised, so that they become a natural resource for you, and harness that power within you. It's alright to have a rest and stop along the way to regain your strength, but just don't stop there for too long!

Maintaining Momentum

You will have come to know yourself and what motivates you, and what doesn't, pretty well by now, but here are a few pointers that will help you to continue on your journey to further self-discovery, and the new goals that you will go on to develop (with your new insight of who you really are):

- **Commitment** – to your goals and yourself - this is an invaluable ally to your continued success. Along with your self-belief, motivation and your willingness to continue to change and experience new things in life.

- **Tenacity** – this is your ability to get up and shake yourself off when you experience a setback. Your determination and persistence to get what you set out to achieve.

- **Learn from What Challenges You** – this is about being objective and learning from what challenges you, and asking yourself why it does so. Keep stepping outside your comfort zone and stretching the boundaries.

- **Take Action** – make things happen for you. Inertia is not a word in your YOU vocabulary!

- **Valuing your Individuality** - It's a stark fact that society has ideas of what we should be doing, should have achieved, what material things we should have, what we should wear, etc., by 'our age' which adds pressure to ourselves to conform to the norms of society.
  You have discovered so much more about yourself since you began your journey towards the YOU that you know that you can be, or already are, so as part of the

maintenance of YOU, you will need to be vigilant to avoid imposing your own stereotypes upon yourself! And remember, age is just that, a number!

- **Accept Yourself** – understand that approval from others isn't necessary for you to achieve your goals and live the life that you want.

- **Mind, Body and Spirit** – Keeping your mind alert with new experiences, setting yourself challenges, getting out there and maintaining your 'Me' time will ensure that these three essentials are actively maintained to provide you with the energy and momentum to keep moving forward to your next horizon.

- **Embracing Uncertainty and Change** – Healthy and productive people tend to be prepared to tolerate a degree of risk and uncertainty in their lives. Demanding certainty in life is a recipe for anxiety and inactivity. Safety comes at a cost – fewer rewards and excitement, fewer new experiences, which is not what YOU are about, so embrace change at every chance you get.

- **Celebrate your Achievements and Successes *every* time** – you really are worth it!

Reflecting on Techniques that worked for you... and techniques that didn't!

Before I introduce you to your final Daily Workout and Visualisation, I would encourage you to reflect on the techniques that you have tried and practised in previous chapters and to reflect on the ones that worked best for you, as well as the ones that didn't (and why). List them below in order of preference:

Daily Workouts and Visualisations I liked

Name	Chapter	Why I liked it and What it helped me with
e.g. The Ring of Motivation & Energy	*e.g. Chapter 1*	

Chapter 6

Daily Workouts and Visualisations that did not work for me

Name	Chapter	Why I liked it and What it helped me with

Now look back to the techniques that didn't work for you and the reasons why. Remember to step outside of your comfort zone here and reflect on your reasons objectively. If you simply found them difficult, you might like to practice them some more, as they may appear different from the last time you tried, with your new found skills and confidence.

And remember you will always have this book to dip into when you want. And of course, for more step-by-step guidance on the various techniques, you can practice with the weblinks until you are proficient.

Daily Workout

Tic Toc Exercise

This is your final Daily Workout and can be useful if you ever get stuck or procrastinate when progressing towards your future goals. This is a technique used in Cognitive Behavioural Therapy (CBT).

TICs are *Task Interfering Cognitions*; the thoughts, attitudes and beliefs that get in the way of your progress. Once you identify these, you need to respond with TOCs, *Task Orienting Cognitions*, which are constructive alternatives to TICs. Are you still with me?

Complete the TIC-TOC table below by following these steps:
1. Identify the goal or task that you want to focus on.
2. In the left hand column (TICs), list your thoughts attitudes and beliefs that get in the way of achieving your aim(s).
3. In the right hand column (TOCs) put responses to all of your TICs that will help you achieve your goal or task.

Goal or Task:	
Task Interfering Cognitions - TICs	**Task Orienting Cognition - TOCs**

Daily Visualisation

The Inner Smile – 'Smile and the world smiles with you' – you have a lot to smile about!

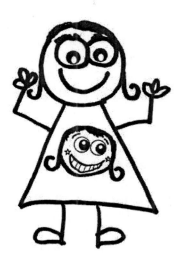

This is an exercise you can use to induce a feeling of wellbeing in yourself, anytime and anywhere, for YOU maintenance.

1. Sit comfortably in any position. Start to become aware of your breathing.
2. Allow a smile to crease the sides of your eyes. Raise the corners of your mouth, ever so slightly.
3. Smile into every part of your body that feels tight or tense, until it begins to relax.
4. Smile into any part of your body that feels especially good. You can increase your smile by expressing gratitude to that part of your body for helping you to stay healthy and strong.

5. Allow the inner smile to reach every corner of your body. Smile into your heart, your lungs, your kidneys, your stomach, etc. Your veins and arteries.
6. Smile into your brain and down your spine, right to the bottom of it.
7. Smile into your life too. Smile and express gratitude for all that you have achieved during your journey to YOU. Smile and express gratitude into your relationships, your health and wellbeing; anything at all.

Notice how the energy around these things begins to shift!

Me Time Meditation

During your 'Me' time in previous chapters of the book, you may have already explored meditation as a way to relax and recuperate your energy. If you haven't tried it before it may feel a bit strange the first time you do it, but keep practising and you will soon begin to feel the benefits. You'll find that you can meditate anywhere and at any time you choose to.

Meditation doesn't necessarily mean sitting cross legged on a mat, with your hands on your knees, chanting. It can be done in any position and at any time that suits you. The benefits of meditation and other mind calming techniques are scientifically validated. When we are awake, our brains produce three types of waves: alpha, beta, and theta. Alpha waves are activated when we are relaxed, but also aware and receptive; they are also associated with pleasurable experiences and with creativity and recall.

Researchers have found that people who meditate regularly have high levels of alpha wave production. Beta waves are activated when our brains are working hard, absorbing information and solving problems. Theta waves are activated when we are drowsy, or feeling emotional.

Meditation is a way of clearing your mind which, when performed regularly, can help to create calmness and confidence. It can recharge the mind, leaving you feeling energised and refreshed.

Having a Go...

To meditate effectively, you need to relax physically first. Find your 'Me' time space where you are comfortable and not likely to be disturbed, then try one of the following two popular methods of relaxation that you may already be familiar with:

1. Close your eyes and become aware of your breathing and repeat some of the breathing exercises in the previous chapters. Imagine a warm feeling of relaxation starting to ebb upwards in your body from your toes, into your ankles and as it progresses up through your body. Relax each body part as the wave of relaxation progresses slowly until it reaches the top of your head. Saying the word 'relax' silently, as you relax each part, also helps.

2. The second method involves visualising yourself somewhere very pleasant and relaxing, like a forest, a beach, or your favourite garden. Keep this picture in your mind, and feel all of the feelings and sensations that go with it. See what you would see, smell what you would smell, hear what you would hear, until you feel relaxed.

   Now focus on your mind and let it fill with space or white light. If a thought intrudes, simply observe it and let it float away. Keep returning your attention to the clear space or white light. Stay like this until you feel well rested. If you find it difficult to focus on space or white light, concentrate on a pool or a restful colour instead.

Some people like to repeat a word or a sound when they meditate. You might like to try 'rest' or 'easy' or 'calm', although this is not obligatory! When you are finished, take your time to get up gently, walk around the room and get your circulation going again with a few stretches.

For more meditation practice and a guided meditation session log on to the website at *www.the-change-coach.co.uk* Alternatively, you could buy or download guided meditation CDs or baroque music, both of which are renowned for increasing the alpha waves in our brain, so conducive to relaxation.

Motivational Quotes

You will have noticed that I have ended each chapter with a motivational quote from a famous or well-known person.

I find that these really work for me. You can get thousands of such quotes to suit all areas and times of your life that can help motivate and lift you, in books or on the internet. I have several, which I change often, stuck on to my goals poster which is displayed on my fridge door, and in other prominent places around me to keep me focused when I get side-tracked or disillusioned!

If these work for you, I'd like to share one that I have in a place that I see every morning. This is attributed to an American theologian, Reinhold Niebuhr, (although authorship is disputed) who included it in a sermon in the 1940s. It has been adapted for use in many 12 step recovery programmes and not being particularly religious myself, I have taken the liberty of adapting it further.

Extended Serenity Prayer

Grant me serenity......
To accept the things I cannot change
Courage to change the things I can
And wisdom - to know the difference.....

Grant me patience for the changes that take time
Appreciation - for ALL that I have
Tolerance - for those with different struggles
And the strength - to get up and try again -
Just one day at a time......

"

Be Happy... NOW!

I've not mentioned happiness on our journey together before
now, as in my mind, happiness is a given and part of who you
are. However, happiness is so important to your whole way of
being; it needs to be covered in this, the last chapter.

Chapter 6

For many people, happiness is conditional. Something just out of reach, and in the future, something they are still searching for. How many people have you heard say "If I win the lottery, I'll ..." or "If I meet my perfect partner, I'll... then I'll be happy"?

Conditional happiness is usually pretty short lived, as there is always something to tweak, change or sort out first.

Have you noticed that so many people are forever in pursuit, looking for that 'something more' that will make them happy or happier than they are now? So long as we continue to aspire or search for happiness, we will always be in the process of becoming happy, rather than being happy now.

There are countless philosophies and books written about the power of living in the 'NOW'. We expend so much of our energy in the search for what we think will make us happy. So it's time to call off the search and give thanks and gratitude for what you already have and for what you have achieved for yourself on your journey to YOU.

Live in the moment instead of striving to reach the next task on your list immediately – savour the moment and enjoy the abundance of what you already have, for a while.

You have had plenty of practice on your journey to challenge your thoughts and change your behaviour. You have made numerous positive choices already and you can also choose to be happy. Whatever events happen in your life, you can make choices to increase (or decrease!) your level of happiness.

Have you noticed that your Energy Radiators seem to lean towards happiness and positivity? That they appear to be naturally and consistently happy despite their lot?

Happiness is indeed a state of mind – you can choose to be happy or not. You have tamed your inner critic and wimp by consistently challenging any negative thoughts already, so you have the capacity to be happier Now. You will have already realised that your positive state of mind propels you more rapidly towards the life that you aspire to.

Your happiness is your responsibility. Don't blame other people if you're not happy. While things around you could change and go bad, it is you who decides how you will respond to them. You can decide to be happy.

Many of your old thought patterns and behaviours will have contributed to your level of happiness. These may have included: self-judgement, complaining, blaming others, dwelling on negative thoughts, obsessing about the past - all will have influenced your previous levels of happiness.

Your new ways of thinking, behaviour and positive attitude will all influence and increase your levels of happiness.

Taking responsibility, being at cause instead of effect, letting go, forgiving yourself and others, and expressing thanks and gratitude, will all contribute to increased levels of happiness and you can choose the level that suits you best. The resources to be happy now are within you already!

Through consistently choosing thoughts and actions which support increased happiness, you also become a powerful magnet for attracting more good into your life, which in turn leads to even more gratitude and increased optimism. A great cycle to be in, don't you think?

Hunter Doherty "Patch" Adams is a renowned American doctor, social activist, and author. Each year he organises a group of volunteers from around the world to travel to various countries where they dress as clowns in an effort to bring humour to orphans, patients, and other people. He uses laughter to heal people and make them feel better. So, as well as adding happiness to your resource bank, throw in some laughter too and hang out with more Energy Radiators and those that make you laugh too.

Chapter 6

With that in mind, here are 10 ideas to finding happiness and laughter in your life:

1. Know yourself

You will be happier as you continue to understand and accept who you are and what makes you tick. Giving yourself regular 'Me' time just to be, and nurturing yourself and your dreams will continue to motivate yourself towards the achievement of your goals and dreams.

2. Count your blessings

There are so many things we should be grateful for, but we often forget them. When you realise and constantly remind yourself how blessed you are, you will certainly be happier. Remember to keep blowing your own trumpet.

3. Accept yourself and find your inner voice

You may have some personality traits that you don't like. For instance, perhaps you are shy and you wish you are an extrovert. Or you wish you were born into a different background. There are many things in life that you just can't control, so just accept yourself as you are. You are unique, and that's something you should be grateful for.

To find true happiness, you must first find your inner voice. Slow down and take some 'Me' time for some inner searching. What will make your life more meaningful? What is true happiness for you? By knowing what your heart says, it will be easier for you to align with it. Listen to your intuition.

4. Continue to challenge yourself

Get used to jumping outside of your comfort zone and challenge any self-limiting beliefs as soon as they pop into your head. Continue to quell that inner critic or wimp into submission. Really go all out for life and grab it. You never know, you may never discover your true passion for something unless you continue to keep giving it a go!

5. Stop comparing yourself with others

Comparing yourself with others won't do you any good. You will either feel proud when you think you are above them, or feel envious and frustrated when you are below. None of that brings true happiness. So stop comparing yourself with others and simply be the best that you know you can be.

6. Spend more quality time with your loved ones

Good relationships can give us happiness more than anything. So spend more quality time with your loved ones, and steer clear of those Moodhoovers and Energy Vampires. In such moments, be sure that you devote your attention to those people you care most about. Remember that some of them won't be around forever and children are only young once.

Let go of the guilt or sense of duty to those individuals that you devoted so much time and attention to in the past.

Continue to review your own life wheel to ensure that your life, and the attention you devote to each area of your life, is constantly in balance.

Chapter 6

7. Keep focused on your goals

Don't allow your goals to become just pieces of paper stuck around your home or work. Keep them colourful and vibrant and continue to take those regular steps to achieving them. Celebrate your achievements regularly – put reminders on your calendar, diary or mobile phone to remind you.

8. Continue to learn and grow as an individual

Continue to nurture your commitment to yourself, your tenacity and persistence to get what you want. Embrace new knowledge and continue to learn from what challenges you, and why. Keep stretching those boundaries and discovering new things – maintain your momentum.

Continue to be your own tourist and get out and explore the world outside your front door and enjoy the simple things in life. Go and get one for yourself!

9. Project yourself

Practice makes perfect as they say, so keep practicing your favourite daily workouts and visualizations. Exude your confident self and keep flaunting your revitalised self-image to the world.

10. Smile

The Law of Attraction states that what you focus on grows. Through focusing on what we don't want, we attract more of the same. So keep focusing on what you do want and continue to grow the good things in life. Remember to water your flowers regularly and keep an eye out for those weeds!

You can beam both your inner and outer smile whenever, and at whoever you choose to. Anytime. Do it regularly. Be Happy NOW!

Time to Look Back... briefly

You have come a long way in such a short time and made profound changes to your attitude, outlook and confidence, which will have all impacted on your goals and the relationships with those around you.

Here is a quick look back and guide to some of the topics that you have tackled along the way and the relevant chapter each topic is from so that you can dip back into it when you need to in the future:

Topic	Chapter Number	Reminder
Self-belief	1	Turn up the gas!
Motivation	1	Put on the Ring of Motivation & Energy.
Self-Discipline	1	Only you can do it.
Willingness to Change and Continue to Challenge yourself	1	Keep stepping out of your comfort zone and notice the huge changes you've already made.
Positive Attitude and Outlook	1 & 2	Stay at 'half full' in your outlook.
Challenge Limiting Beliefs	2	Keep asking yourself those internal questions of why you think this about something.

Cause not Effect	2	Stay at Cause *not* Effect (unless you choose). That's not being defeatist but on occasion, you may be at effect as you have been the instigator of the Cause; e.g. achieving your goals and being where you want to be.
Your inner critic or wimp	2	Keep your inner critic or wimp in check and dismiss those doubts as soon as they pop up in your head.
Moodhoovers and Energy Vampires	2	Keep clear of them. Keep the company of positive people. Aspire to be an Energy Radiator but don't let yourself get drained by allowing others to become dependent on you to offload their complaining.
Life Wheel	3	Revisit your Wheel of Life or Life Wheel frequently and check the amount of attention you are giving to the important areas of your life are still in balance. Also check whether the important areas need updating, as different areas become more important to you as you continue to develop personally.

Goals	4	Continue to monitor (and celebrate) progress towards the achievement of your goals. Refine them, set new ones.
Self-Image	5	Revisit your Top to Toe image audit occasionally to check if it needs updating as you continue to develop towards the YOU that you set out to be. Remember your individuality and that age is just a number.
ME Time	All	This should be a regular habit for you now, so keep doing it and exploring and embracing new experiences.

Looking Backwards and Moving Forwards

This is your final time to reflect in the book, although I hope you are much more reflective now that you have had so much practice!

Do continue to reflect regularly, as this will help you to learn from events in your life that sometimes do not go exactly as you planned, and to learn and plan to be more effective in everything you do in the future.

Use the space below to reflect on all the positive changes you have made on your journey to YOU and also the things that

Chapter 6

challenged you most (and why). Then go one step further and think about the reasons certain things challenged you and whether you need to include the learning from these into your future goals.

Positive changes	Things that challenged me most and why

Daily Checklist - YOU

Tick these off as you achieve and practice them:

Completed the like/dislike exercise	
Practiced my Daily Workout	
Practiced my Daily Visualisation	
Researched motivational quotes that work for me	
Practiced 'Me' time Meditation	
Reflected on my journey to YOU	
Added contacts to my Personal Resource Bank	

Summary

Well, here we are! The final stage of your journey of self-discovery back to YOU. Or is it really the final stage?

Your continued success is about deciding what you want, working out what's important to you and then going out and grabbing it. You can achieve whatever you want - you just need to go after it. Do it for the right reasons – be true to yourself.

You have learned so much about yourself on your journey to YOU that being true to the real you, shouldn't be difficult. Be positive and optimistic about your chances of success. The more you believe in yourself, the better you will be able to sell yourself. It will show in your face, your posture, body language and your confidence. Learn how to ask for things in the way that is most likely to achieve the best results for YOU. Think it out beforehand, planning and rehearsing is pivotal to the successful outcome that you want. Remember to practice, use the techniques in the workbook (and on the weblinks) to your advantage.

Your new attitude and behaviours will all contribute to your continued success in being the YOU that you set out to be. Continuing focused hard work is one of the keys to this success, so keep your eyes on your goals and continue taking the next steps towards completing them. Once there, develop new challenges for yourself.

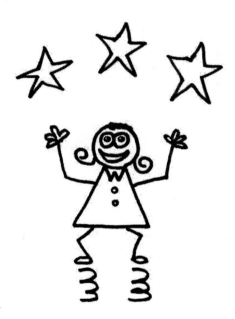

If you get stuck or find yourself at a crossroads, dip into your resource bank to inspire you. If you are still unsure which way to do something, seek out your trusted friends for objective advice.

Tackle the issue both ways and see what works best for you. Remember it's all about YOU and what suits you best. Focus your conscious mind on things you desire or want, not those that you fear – dream big!

There is a Neuro Linguistic Programming (NLP) pre-supposition that *'There is no failure, only feedback'*. You have already explored what challenges you in this and previous chapters, so when you get knocked back, try not to take it personally, get back up there, learn from it and do it again, but tackle it differently!

So pursue excellence with optimism in all that you do, enjoy the experience.

I wish you every success and happiness, on your continued journey to your next horizon,

Best wishes always,

Lynne

www.the-change-coach.co.uk

"

If you don't get lost, there's a chance YOU may never be found.

Author Unknown

"

CPSIA information can be obtained at www.ICGtesting.com
Printed in the USA
LVOW10s1139270116

471830LV00021B/546/P